The Ketogenic Vegan Cookbook

More Than 50 Delicious Vegan Recipes for Your Ketogenic Diet

By

Elisa Hayes

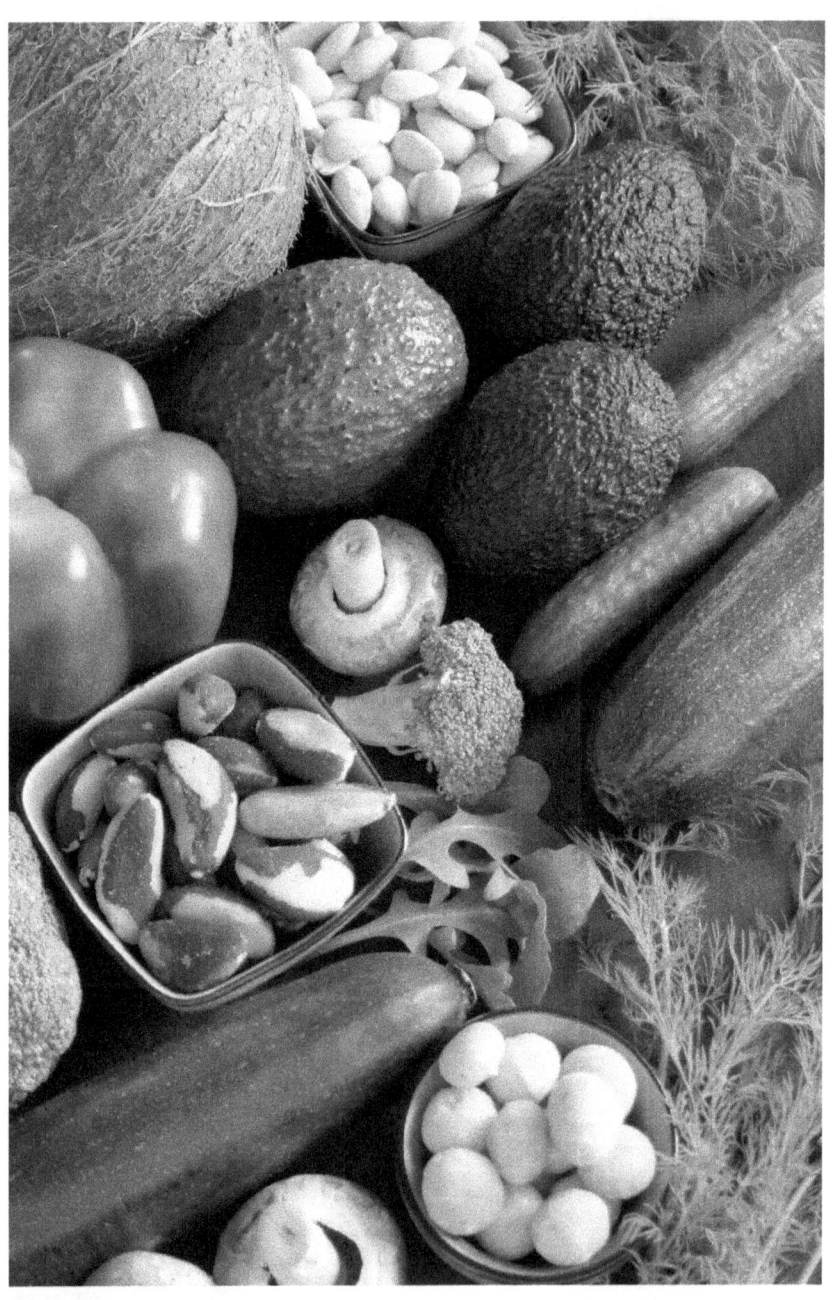

Table of Contents

Introduction 7
- PESTO SPAGHETTI WITH ZUCCHINI (ZOODLES) 11
- CAULIFLOWER MUSHROOM RISOTTO 14
- CAULIFLOWER STEAKS 17
- EVERYDAY LEMON TAHINI 18
- KALE TOFU STIR FRY 20
- VEGAN KETO WALNUT CHILI 21
- AIR FRYER BUFFALO CAULIFLOWER WINGS 23
- GRAIN FREE GRANOLA 25
- KETO PEANUT BUTTER RAMEN 26
- CURRY CABBAGE 28
- VEGAN ZUCCHINI PASTA ALFREDO 31
- VEGAN QUICHE MUGS 33
- CURRIED TOMATO SOUP 34
- LEMON TURMERIC ROASTED CAULIFLOWER 36
- LEMON BRUSSELS SPROUTS WITH GARLIC 37
- SIMPLE VEGAN BOK CHOY SOUP 39
- BAKED TOFU FRIES 40
- CAULIFLOWER MUSHROOM RISOTTO 43
- SILKY VEGAN CAULIFLOWER SOUP 45
- VEGETARIAN RED CURRY STIR FRY 48
- CREAMY CAULIFLOWER GARLIC RICE 50
- HEALTHY CAULIFLOWER FRIED RICE 52
- MEXICAN CAULIFLOWER RICE BURRITO BOWL 55
- CAULIFLOWER FIESTA RICE SALAD 57
- CURRIED CAULIFLOWER RICE KALE SOUP 59
- PESTO CAULIFLOWER RICE 61
- BLISSFUL BASIL SWEET POTATOES 63
- SUSHI VEGAN CAULIFLOWER RICE 67

SPANISH CAULIFLOWER RICE	69
FRITTERS WITH CHIPOTLE LIME AIOLI	70
CAULIFLOWER BIBIMBAP	73
ROASTED BOK CHOY	75
VEGAN SHAKSHUKA	77
REFRIGERATED VEGETABLE SALAD	80
GINGER, SESAME, WALNUT AND HEMP SEED LETTUCE WRAPS	82
ROASTED PEPPERS AND ONIONS	84
CURRY PUMPKIN SOUP	86
TOFU PERFECT BAKED CRISPY	88
KETO CAULIFLOWER STUFFING	90
KETO VEGAN PIZZA STICKS	92
ZUCCHINI NOODLES WITH AVOCADO SAUCE	93
VEGAN TOFU BUFFALO WINGS	95
CAULIFLOWER RICE PILAF WITH HEMP SEED	97
GRILLED GARLIC CAULIFLOWER	99
MASHED TURNIPS	100
ENSALADA TALONG – FILIPINO EGGPLANT SALAD	102
KETO MASHED POTATOES	104

© Copyright 2021 by Elisa Hayes - All rights reserved.

The following Book is reproduced below with the goal of providing information that is as accurate and reliable as possible. Regardless, purchasing this Book can be seen as consent to the fact that both the publisher and the author of this book are in no way experts on the topics discussed within and that any recommendations or suggestions that are made herein are for entertainment purposes only. Professionals should be consulted as needed prior to undertaking any of the action endorsed herein.

This declaration is deemed fair and valid by both the American Bar Association and the Committee of Publishers Association and is legally binding throughout the United States.

Furthermore, the transmission, duplication, or reproduction of any of the following work including specific information will be considered an illegal act irrespective of if it is done electronically or in print. This extends to creating a secondary or tertiary copy of the work or a recorded copy and is only allowed with the express written consent from the Publisher. All additional rights reserved.

The information in the following pages is broadly considered a truthful and accurate account of facts and as such, any inattention, use, or misuse of the information in question by the reader will render any resulting actions solely under their purview. There are no scenarios in which the publisher or the original author of this work can be in any fashion deemed liable for any hardship or damages that may befall them after undertaking information described herein.

Additionally, the information in the following pages is intended only for informational purposes and should thus be thought of as universal. As befitting its nature, it is presented without assurance regarding its prolonged validity or interim quality. Trademarks that are mentioned are done without written consent and can in no way be considered an endorsement from the trademark holder.

Introduction

The path to a perfect body and good physical health was very thorny for me. The only one wish which I was making for my birthdays for many years was to be a slim and beautiful girl. Alas, everything can't be as in fairy tales and the miracle didn't happen; my mirror was still showing the same fat, pimple girl. In childhood, the problem of being overweight didn't bother me much; I can say that I didn't care about it at all, I didn't know that weight would be momentous for me. I was an ordinary smiling child, playing with my peers, going to school, and traveling with my parents. That time my chubby cheeks seemed very sweet to everyone. But that was then. At 11-year-old, I went to middle school. New people, new teachers, I had no friends at all. Mentally I was broken. I counted the minutes until the end of the last lesson, to quickly sit in my mom's car and leave school. I started to eat a lot. Now I see that in this way I am stressed, but then the food served as my antidepressant. Dozens of hamburgers, fried potatoes, coke – they were "my best friends". In addition to everything, I started to have horrible skin problems, it seemed to me that there was no place on my face wherever they hadn't appeared yet. Time passed and I no longer loved my reflection in the mirror even in 1%. I couldn't wear the clothes that I liked. I usually wore oversized shorts and t-shirts. I couldn't afford to wear a short dress and high heels. At 15-year-old I weighed more than 270lbs. I remember what I felt in those days, as it is happening now. I felt anger, irritation, hatred, and self-loathing. That prom party was the most terrible day of my life. Thank God it's over!

In those years, the keto diet was not very popular, fasting and drinking diets (which, as you already know, did not help me much) were more popular. Perhaps I wouldn't do anything, but my health problems were becoming more serious. It seemed that my body was simply screaming: please help me!

I remember the day that changed my life on a dime. I came to the clinic with pain in my stomach. But this time, I not only received painkillers but also found a mentor and friend. This was my physician. She had examined me and recommended that I go on a diet. I didn't want to do something and was categorically against it. However, my mind changed when she said: love your body, care about it, and it will thank you. What was my surprise when the diet turned out to be very simple to follow. Is it so easy to love myself? As you could understand I am talking about my favorite keto diet. Every day I was eating a maximum of proteins and a minimum of carbohydrates. That meant to consume meat, poultry, and fish and make restrictions for vegetables, fruits, and sweets. After 2 weeks, I lost 83lbs, and further results were getting better and better. All this time I was under the supervision of a doctor and this yielded results. A year later, I completely changed all the clothes in my wardrobe and oh my God I was able to wear a short dress and skirts! Now I can say that I am the happiest person. It happened because I fell in love with myself and started treating my body as a diamond. My life was filled with bright colors, I have a beloved husband, children, work, friends, I am healthy and like myself in the mirror. I am telling this story to prove that the right diet can solve almost all problems with body and health. It is a fact that our body is capable of dealing with dramatic changes, it is only worth loving it. Never rest on your laurels, never give up and forbid people to say that you cannot do something. You are already a great fellow that you bought this cookbook and decided to take a step ahead in the direction to your dream. Let this book become your ray of hope, a lifesaver on the way to your wonderful transformation. If you believe in yourself and love your body, believe me, the result won't be long in coming. You will see in the mirror a completely new version of yourself, updated physically and mentally! Just trust the keto diet and your inner voice. Set a goal today and start the way of achieving it right now. Don't try to do it all in one time; let it be a small step day by day. Exactly now, this is the right time to start creating a new version of you. If this diet was able to change my life, I'm sure it will help you too!

PESTO SPAGHETTI WITH ZUCCHINI (ZOODLES)

Ingredients

- 2 medium-sized zucchini, spiral-shaped (see notes below)
- ⅓ cup vegan pesto, + more if necessary
- ½ red onion, finely sliced and cut in half
- 6 mushrooms, thinly sliced (cremini or white bud)
- 10 cherry tomatoes, cut in half
- 2 garlic cloves, finely chopped
- 2 tsp olive oil
- salt to taste
- freshly ground black pepper (optional)
- chopped red pepper (optional)
- cashew cream (optional drizzle)

Instructions

1. In a skillet, heat the olive oil over medium to high heat.
2. Add chopped garlic, chopped onions, and chopped mushrooms. Add about ¼ tsp salt.
3. Bake until vegetables are tender and soft, but crisp. Keep in mind that the water is cooked when the mushrooms are cooked. Put aside.
4. Quickly clean the pan with a damp towel.

5. Heat ¼ cup pesto, add the zucchini spaghetti in a spiral shape, and cook for 1 to 2 min over medium heat to cook quickly.

6. Add fried onions/mushrooms and halves of cherry tomatoes.

7. Add the rest of the pesto. If necessary, you can add more pesto than the amount indicated above. (optional) Add a dash of cream if using it.

8. Cook another 1 to 2 min, stirring regularly.

9. Season with salt freshly ground black pepper and crushed red pepper (if used).

Prep time: 10 min; **Servings:** 3

Macros: Cal 226n Cal from Fat 176 Fat 19.6g Saturated Fat 1.9g Carbs 11.4g Fiber 3.1g Sugar 6.3g Protein 4.5g

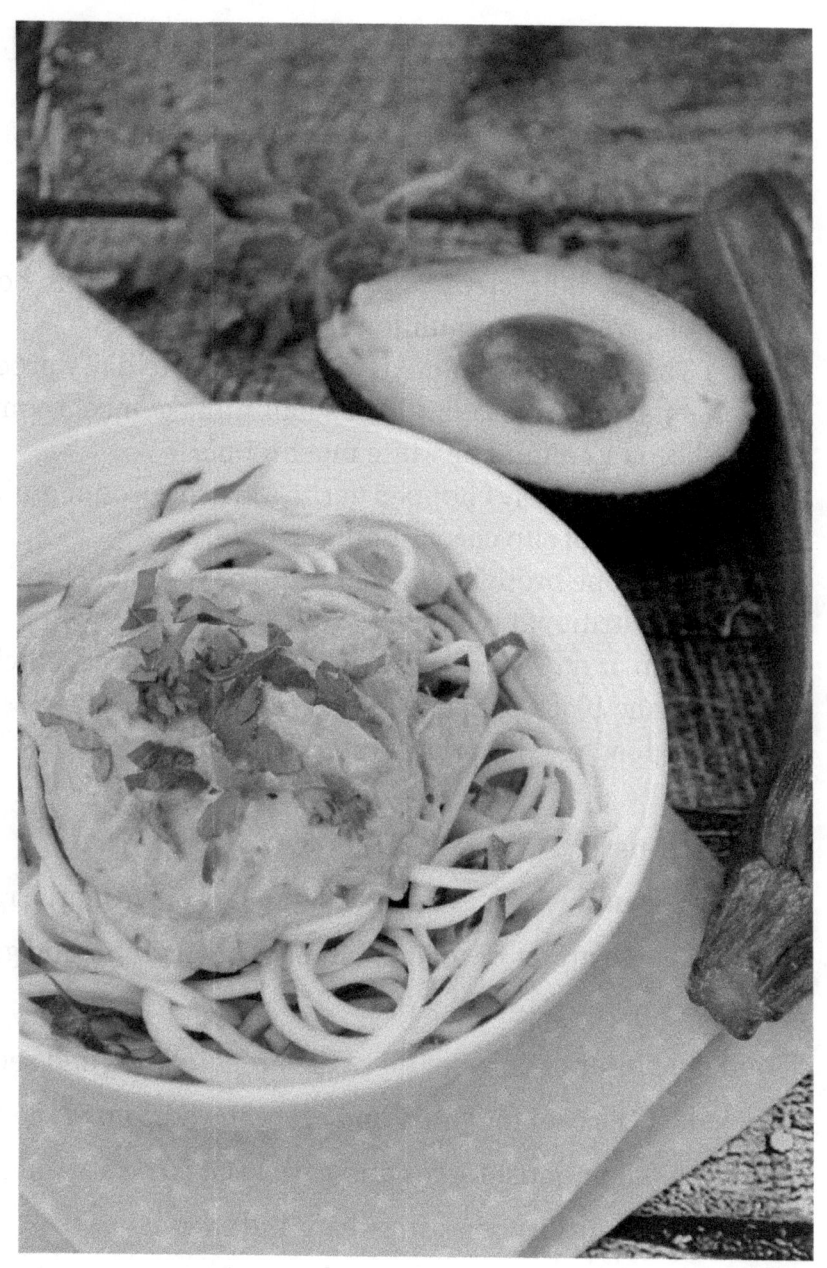

CAULIFLOWER MUSHROOM RISOTTO

Ingredients

- 1 cup medium-sized gold cauliflower 4-5 cups pre-cooked fresh gold frozen cauliflower
- 1 Tbsp coconut oil for AIP or sensitivity to dairy products, 1 small onion, diced, 1 lb of small shiitake mushrooms, sliced or cremini or white mushrooms
- 3 cloves oFinely chopped garlic, 2 Tbsp coconut amino acids, 1 full cup coconut milk
- 1 cup bone broth or chicken broth or vegetable broth, ¼ cup nutritional yeast
- ½ tsp or more sea salt, to taste, 2 Tbsp tapioca starch
- Ground black pepper to taste (skip for AIP)
- Chopped parsley to decorate

Instructions

1. Remove cauliflower leaves and cut the flowers from the roots.
2. Use a cheese grater or food processor with a grater and grated cauliflower to the size of the rice.
3. Add the butter or coconut oil to the prepared pan and set it to "Sautéed." Let's cool for 5 min and cover the bottom of the pan.
4. Add the onion, mushrooms and garlic and cook, stirring, for 7 min, until the mushrooms are sweaty and soft.
5. Add the coconut amino acids and sauté for 5 min until the vegetables are brown. Turn off the instant pot.

6. Add the cauliflower rice and coconut milk. bone broth, nutritional yeast, and sea salt. Stir together.

7. Close the lid, make sure the valve is closed and set the instant pot to "Manual" for 2 min

8. Release the pressure valve and open the lid.

9. Sprinkle tapioca starch on the risotto and stir until thickened. Add more salt if you wish. Add ground black pepper if you are using it.

10. Serve hot, sprinkled with parsley chopped.

Prep time: 15 min; **Servings:** 4

Macros: Cal 299.05 Cal from Fat 172 Fat 19.15g Saturated Fat 15.12g Cholesterol 9.6mg Sodium 546.4mg Carbs 27.61g Fiber 8.31g Sugar 8.64g Protein 10.62g

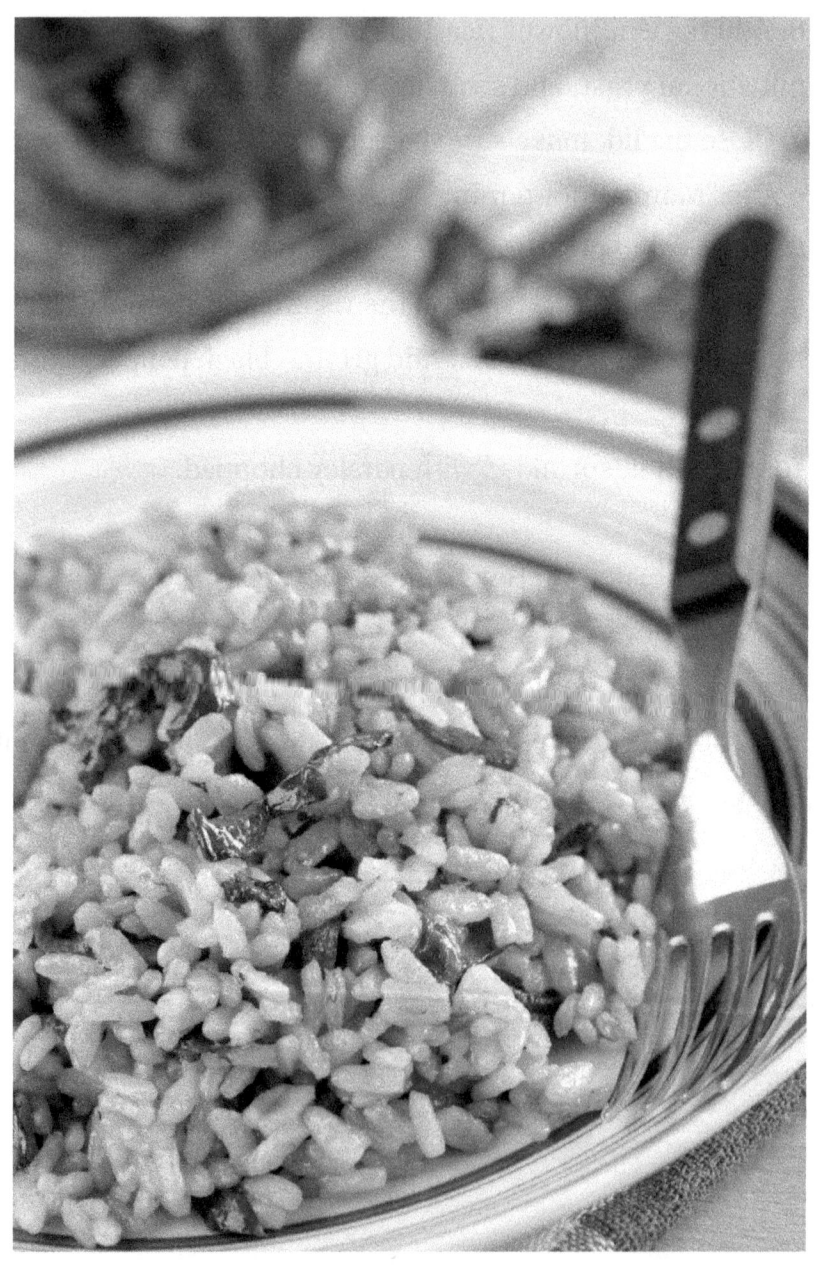

CAULIFLOWER STEAKS

Ingredients

- 1 big cauliflower
- 3 Tbsp split olive oil
- ¼ cup parsley chopped
- ¼ cup chopped raw pumpkin seeds
- Pink Himalayan salt to taste
- black pepper to taste

Instructions

1. Preheat the oven to 400° C and line a baking sheet with parchment paper.
2. Cut the cauliflower stalk to rest on a flat surface. The number oFillets depends on the size and condition of the cauliflower.
3. Place the cauliflower on the baking sheet coated and sprinkle with 2 Tbsp olive oil. Sprinkle the salt with a pinch of salt and pepper. Bake for 30 min or until cauliflower is golden.
4. While cooking cauliflower, mix remaining Tbsp of olive with parsley and pumpkin seeds and season with salt and pepper. When the cauliflower is ready to fry, for the right amount of tahini lemon vinaigrette and cover it with the spice mixture.

Prep time: 5 min; **Servings:** 2-4
Macros: Cal 350 Carbs 50 g Fat 7 g Protein 22 g

EVERYDAY LEMON TAHINI

Ingredients

- ¼ cup + 1 Tbsp lukewarm filtered water
- ¼ cup tahini
- 1 garlic clove, diced
- 2 Tbsp lemon juice
- ½ tsp maple syrup
- ¼ tsp pink Himalayan salt
- A pinch of of black pepper

Instructions

1. Mix all ingredients in a blender
2. Blender until smooth

Prep time: 5 min; **Servings:** 6

Macros: Cal 140 Carbs 4g Fat 11g Protein 8g

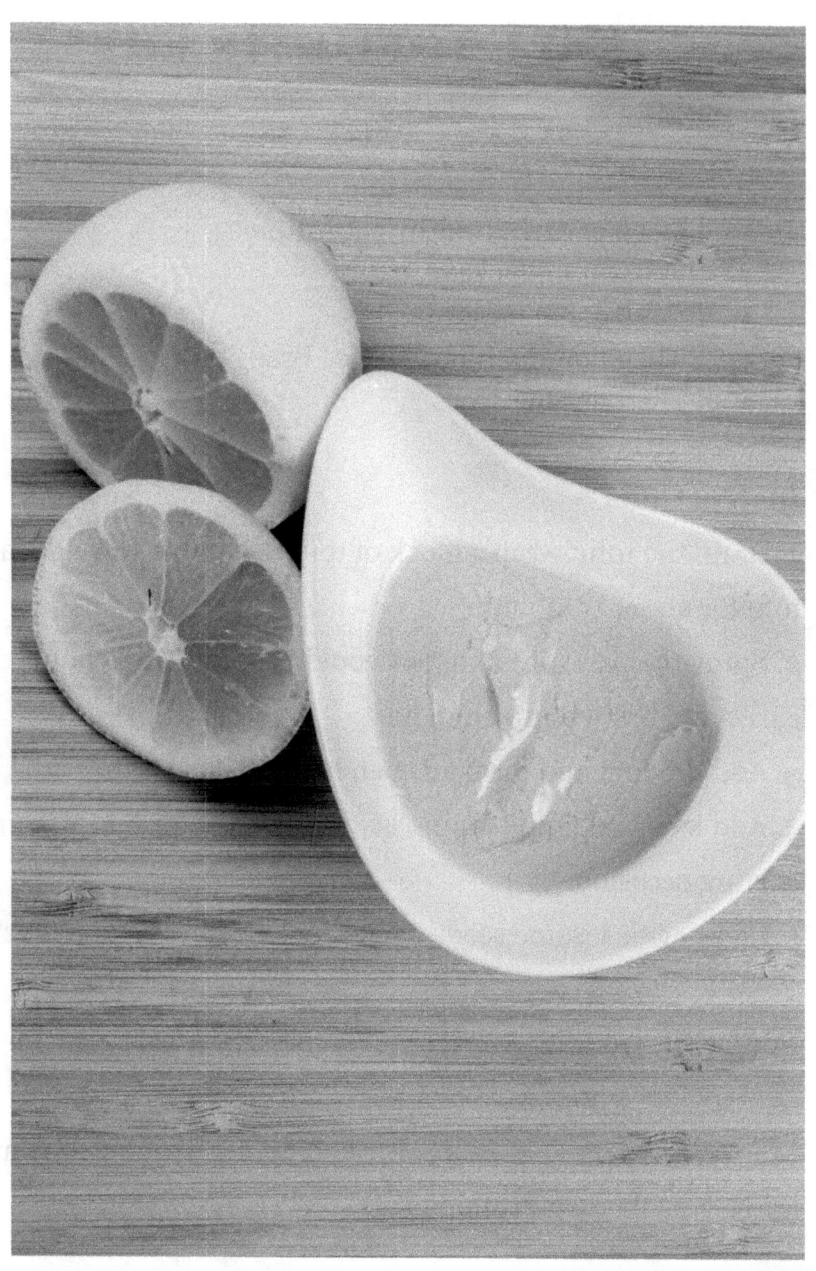

KALE TOFU STIR FRY

Ingredients

- 1 block of extra healthy cubic tofu
- 6 cups chopped kale
- 1 clove garlic minced
- 2 Tbsp liquid amino acids of Bragg or soy sauce
- 1 Tbsp sesame seeds

Instructions

1. Drain the tofu: wrap a block of tofu in a paper towel. Drain the tofu for about 15-20 min
2. Spray the pan with nonstick cooking spray. Add chopped garlic and bring to medium heat.
3. Add the tofu and form an even layer. Bake 2 min
4. Add kale and liquid amino acids and cook for 8 to 10 minutes, stirring occasionally.
5. Cover with sesame seeds and enjoy!

Prep time: 10 min; **Servings:** 3

Macros: Cal 232 Fat 12 g Saturated fat 2 g Sodium 1001 mg Carbs 7 g Fiber 6 g Protein 26 g

VEGAN KETO WALNUT CHILI

Ingredients

- 2 Tbsp extra virgin olive oil
- 5 thinly sliced celery stalks 2 garlic cloves, finely chopped 1 ½ tsp ground cinnamon
- 2 tsp chili powder 4 tsp ground cumin
- 1½ smoked pepper tsp 2 large pickled chipotle peppers
- 2 finely chopped green peppers
- 2 diced zucchini
- 8 g of chopped mushrooms in a food processor 1 ½ Tbsp tomato puree 1 can of 15 oz tomato cubes 3 cups of water ½ cup coconut milk 2½ cups grated soy meat
- 1 cup chopped raw walnuts
- Tbsp unsweetened cocoa powder
- Salt and pepper to taste
  To serve:
- 2 Tbsp fresh coriander leaves
- 1 sliced avocado
- 2 Tbsp sliced radish.

Instructions

1. Heat the oil in a large saucepan over medium heat. Add celery and cook for 4 min Add garlic, cinnamon, chili powder, cumin, and pepper and stir until fragrant, about 2 minutes more.

2. Add pepper, zucchini, mushrooms, and cook for 5 min

3. Add the chipotle, tomato puree, tomatoes, water, coconut milk, soy meat, nuts, and cocoa powder. Reduce heat to medium-low and simmer for about 20-25 min until thickened and vegetables are tender.

4. Season with salt and pepper. Cover with avocado, radish, and coriander.

Prep time: 10 min; **Servings:** 4

Macros: Cal 353

AIR FRYER BUFFALO CAULIFLOWER WINGS

Ingredients

- 3-4 Tbsp hot sauce
- 1 Tbsp almond flour
- 1 Tbsp avocado oil
- Salt to taste
- 1 medium-sized cauliflower, washed and thoroughly dried

Instructions

1. Preheat the fryer to 400° F.
2. Mix hot sauce, almond flour, avocado oil, and salt in a large bowl.
3. Add the cauliflower and mix until covered.
4. Put half of the cauliflower in the fryer and cook for 12 to 15 min (or until it is crisp on the edges with a small cock or reaches the desired level).
5. Be sure to open the fryer and shake the fry basket halfway to rotate the cauliflower. Delete and book.
6. Add the second portion, but cook 2 to 3 min less.

Prep time: 5 min; **Servings:** 4

Macros: Cal 48 | Carbs 1 g | Fat 4 g Sodium 265 mg | Potassium 94 mg Vitamin A: 15 IU | Vitamin C: 20.2 mg | Calcium: 10 mg Iron: 0.2 mg

GRAIN FREE GRANOLA

Ingredients

- 1 cup nuts and seeds
- 1 Tbsp agave syrup or sweetener of your choice
- ½ tsp vanilla extract
- 1 tsp almond extract
- 1 Tbsp melted coconut oil
- ¼ cup coconut chips

Instructions

1. Preheat the oven to 325° F.
2. Mix the agave syrup, extract vanilla, almond extract, and coconut oil in a bowl. Microwave 20-30 seconds to combine.
3. For the mixture over the nuts and seeds (no coconut chips) and mix well. Bake for 10 min. Return and cook for 5 min Add the coconut chips and cook for another 5 min.

Prep time: 10 min; **Servings:** 4

Macros: Cal 299 | Carbs 14 g Protein 6g Fat 25 g Saturated Fat 8 g Cholesterol 0 mg Sodium 6 mg Potassium 243 mg Fiber 4 g Sugar 4g Calcium: 25 mg Iron: 1.5 mg

KETO PEANUT BUTTER RAMEN

Ingredients

Sweet and spicy peanut sauce

- ¼ cup all-natural peanut butter (no added sugar, crisp or fresh)
- 1 tsp sambal oelek (add more if you like spicy)
- 1 ½ Tbsp soy sauce
- 1 tsp Truvia or another sugar-free sweetener that you like

Noodles and toppings

- 1 pack of House Foods Shirataki noodles
- 1 block of extra healthy tofu (about 100 g)
- 1 Tbsp coconut oil
- 1-2 chopped green onions
- 1 chopped cayenne pepper
- sesame seed drizzle (optional)

Instructions

1. Cut the tofu into large cubes and heat the frying pan over medium heat. Add the coconut oil (1 Tbsp) and add it to the tofu. Stir so that the tofu does not stick. Once the tofu starts to turn a bit brown, turn it on with more soy sauce and stir. Remove the fire and reserve. You want the tofu to have a crispy exterior, but a sweet center.

2. Boil water (2 cups are enough). While the water boils, put the peanut butter (4 Tbsp) in a large bowl with the sambal oelek (chili paste), soy sauce (1 Tbsp) and the Truvia (1 tsp)).

3. Slowly add ⅓ cup boiled water into the large bowl. Mix well to emulsify. Depending on how you are, you may need a little more hot water or less. You are looking for a sauce that is neither thick nor liquid.

4. Remove the noodles from the package and place it in the microwave for 2 min Add the noodles to the peanut sauce and mix. When combined, sesame seeds, soy sauce, and chopped cayenne pepper.

Prep time: 10 min; **Servings:** 1

Macros: Cal 574 | Carbs 13.5 g | Protein 23 g | Fat 49 g | Saturated Fat 15.5 g Fiber 9 g

CURRY CABBAGE

Ingredients

- 1 lb of green cabbage, washed
- 2 Tbsp oil coconut or ¼ cup water/vegetable broth
- ½ cup chopped onion
- 2 garlic cloves, finely chopped
- 1 tsp ground coriander 1 tsp ground turmeric 1 tsp dried thyme leaves or 2 sprigs oFresh thyme
- ½ tsp cumin 1 chopped carrot
- 1-14 g of coconut milk ½ cup water 3/4 tsp sea salt, or to taste

Instructions

1. Cut cabbage into strips 1 inch thick, set aside in a bowl.

2. Heat the oil in a large saucepan over medium heat.

3. Add the onion and garlic and cook until tender, stirring for about 3 min

4. Add coriander, turmeric, thyme, caraway, carrot, cabbage, and stir. Add cocoon milk, water, and boil.

5. Cover the pan and simmer and cook for about 20 min or until the sauce thickens.

6. Delicious served with brown rice or baked potatoes and a salad!

Prep time: 10 min; **Servings:** 4

Macros: Macros: 171 / 715 kJ Fat 13 g Protein 3 g Carbohydrate: 12 g

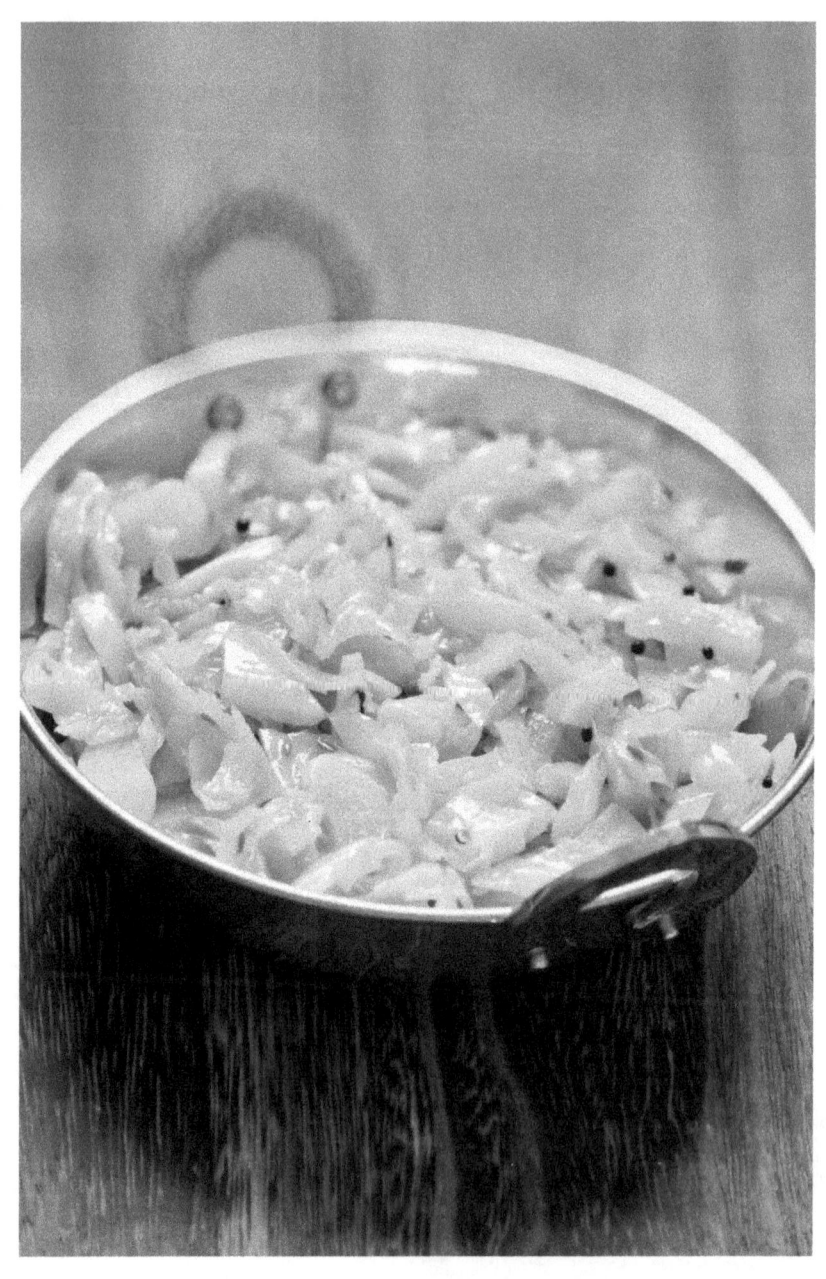

VEGAN ZUCCHINI PASTA ALFREDO

Ingredients

- 2 medium-sized spiral zucchini
- 1-2 TB vegan parmesan (optional)
- Quick Alfredo sauce
- Soak ½ cup raw water for a few hours or 10 min in boiling water • 2 Tbsp of lemon juice
- Nutritional yeast 3 TB
- 2 tsp white miso
- 1 tsp onion powder
- ½ tsp garlic powder
- ¼ to ½ cup water

Instructions

1. Zucchini noodles spiral.

2. Add all ingredients in a blender (starting with ¼ cup water) and mix until smooth. If your sauce is too thick, add 1 more Tbsp water.

3. Cover the zucchini noodles with Alfredo sauce and, if desired, a vegan parmesan.

Prep time: 5 min; **Servings:** 6
Macros: Cal 225 Cal from fat 144 Fat 16 g Carbs 19 g Fiber 6 g Protein 14 g

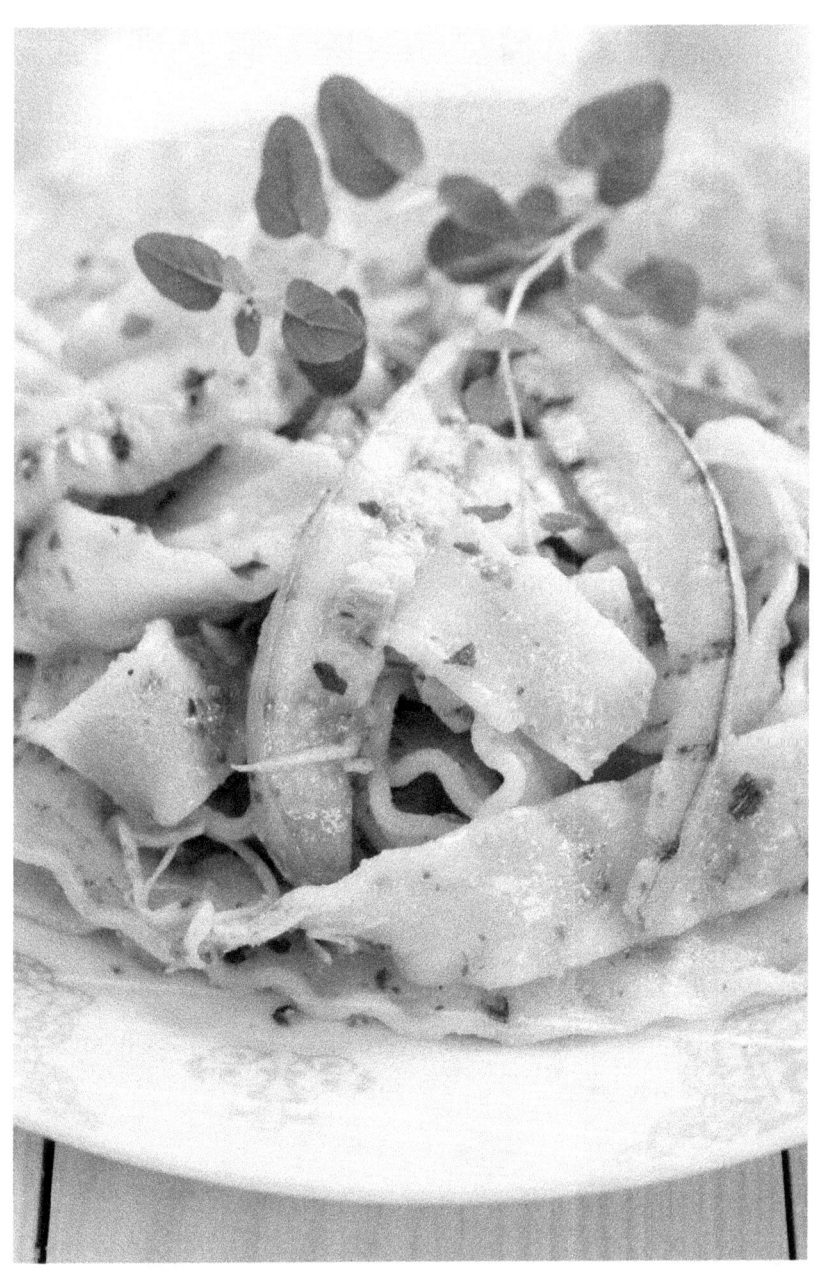

VEGAN QUICHE MUGS

Ingredients

- 1 extra stable tofu block (14 oz)
- 3 Tbsp water
- 1 Tbsp tomato sauce
- 2 Tbsp Dijon mustard
- 1 Tbsp lemon juice
- 1 Tbsp corn flour
- ½ cup nutritional yeast
- 2 tsp garlic herbs

Instructions

1. Preheat the oven to 350° F, cover the muffin pan with nonstick mussels or spray with nonstick cooking spray and set aside.
2. Mix all ingredients except green leafy vegetables in a blender and blend until smooth. Add more water if necessary, to facilitate mixing.
3. For the contents of the blender into a large mixing bowl, add green leafy vegetables and stir.
4. Spoon in the form of a muffin.
5. Bake for 30 to 35 min or until the edges begin to brown.

Prep time: 10 min; **Servings:** 12
Macros: Cal 57 Cal from fat 18 Fat 2 g Carbs 5 g Fiber 2 g Protein 6 g

CURRIED TOMATO SOUP

Ingredients

- 28 oz (800 g) chopped fresh tomatoes
- 1/5 cup (150 g) of cauliflower flowers
- 4 onions (chopped onions), finely chopped
- 1 Tbsp sweet curry powder
- 1 tsp ginger puree
- 1 tsp garlic puree
- 2 cups (500 mL) warm vegetable broth
- salt and pepper

Instructions

1. Add all the ingredients to the slow cooker and mix.
2. Cover and cook at high temperature for 3 hours.
3. Let the tomatoes cool for a while, then mash it in a blender, adjust the herbs, and serve.

Prep time: 5 min; **Servings:** 4

Macros: Cal 54 | Carbs 12 g | Protein 2g | Sodium 758 mg Potassium 457 mg | Fiber 3g | Sugar 6g

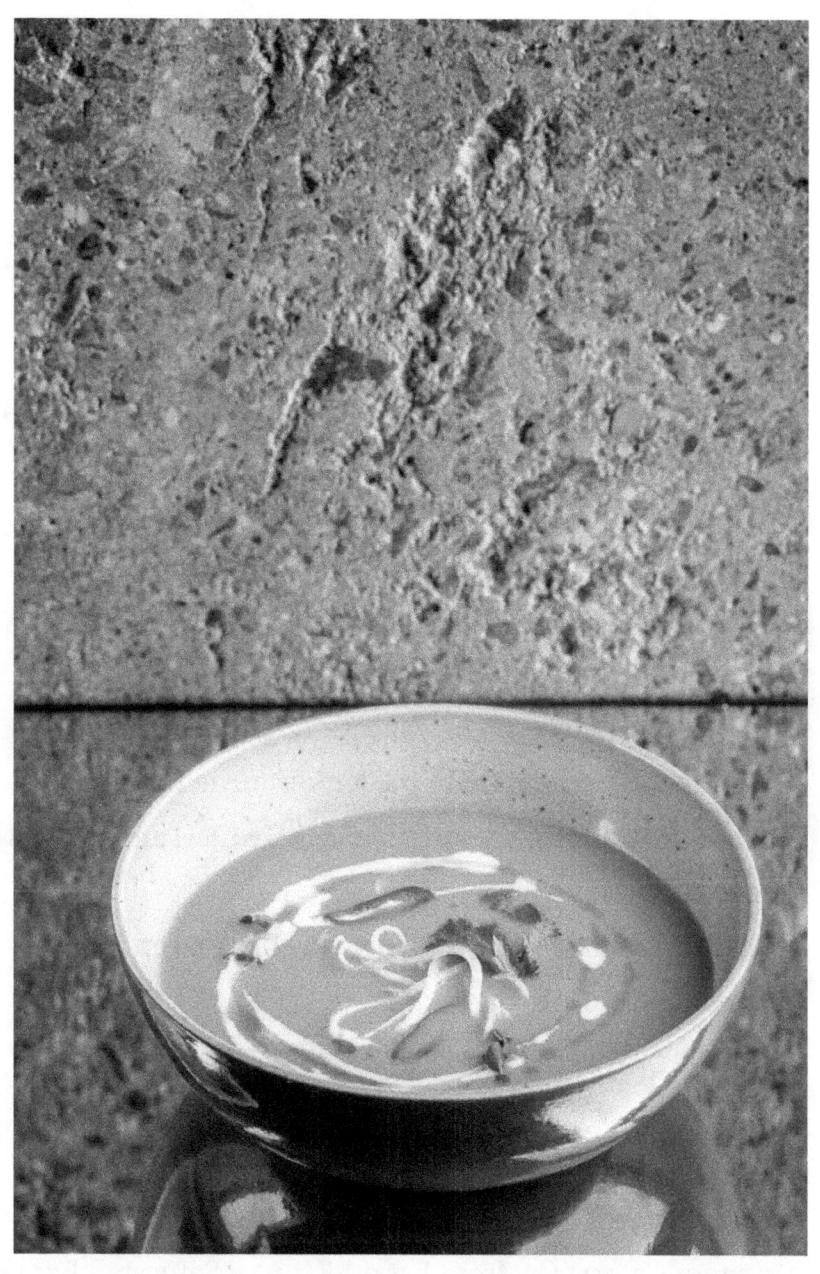

LEMON TURMERIC ROASTED CAULIFLOWER

Ingredients

- 1 cup cauliflower
- 2 Tbsp chopped parsley
- Lemon and turmeric vinaigrette
- 3 Tbsp avocado oil
- 2 Tbsp lemon juice
- 3 cloves of garlic, finely chopped
- 1 tsp turmeric powder
- ½ tsp sea salt

Instructions

1. Preheat the oven to 425 F.
2. Chop the cauliflower into bite-size bunches.
3. Beat the ingredients with the lemon-turmeric vinaigrette.
4. Place the cauliflower flowers in a large bowl and mix with the vinaigrette.
5. Spread cauliflower on a baking sheet in 1 layer.
6. Roast in the oven for 20-25 min
7. Sprinkle with chopped parsley before serving.

Prep time: 5 min; **Servings:** 4

Macros: Cal 107 Cal from Fat 90 Fat 10 g Saturated Fat 1 g Carbs 3 g

LEMON BRUSSELS SPROUTS WITH GARLIC

Ingredients

- 2 cups of Brussels sprouts
- 3-5 cloves of garlic
- 1 Tbsp avocado oil
- salt + pepper to taste

Instructions

1. Preheat the oven to 400° F.
2. Wash and dry the sprouts.
3. Cut in half and loose outer leaves.
4. Place them directly on a baking sheet.
5. Cut the garlic cloves and cut into large pieces.
6. Mix the sprouts and garlic with avocado oil, salt, and pepper.
7. Bake for 15 min, then stir sprouts and garlic.
8. Cook another 15 to 20 min (the total cooking time depends on the size of your sprouts).

Prep time: 7 min; **Servings:** 2

Macros: Cal 106 | Carbs 9 g | Protein 3g | Fat 7 g Saturated Fat 1 g Fiber 3 g | Sugar 1 g

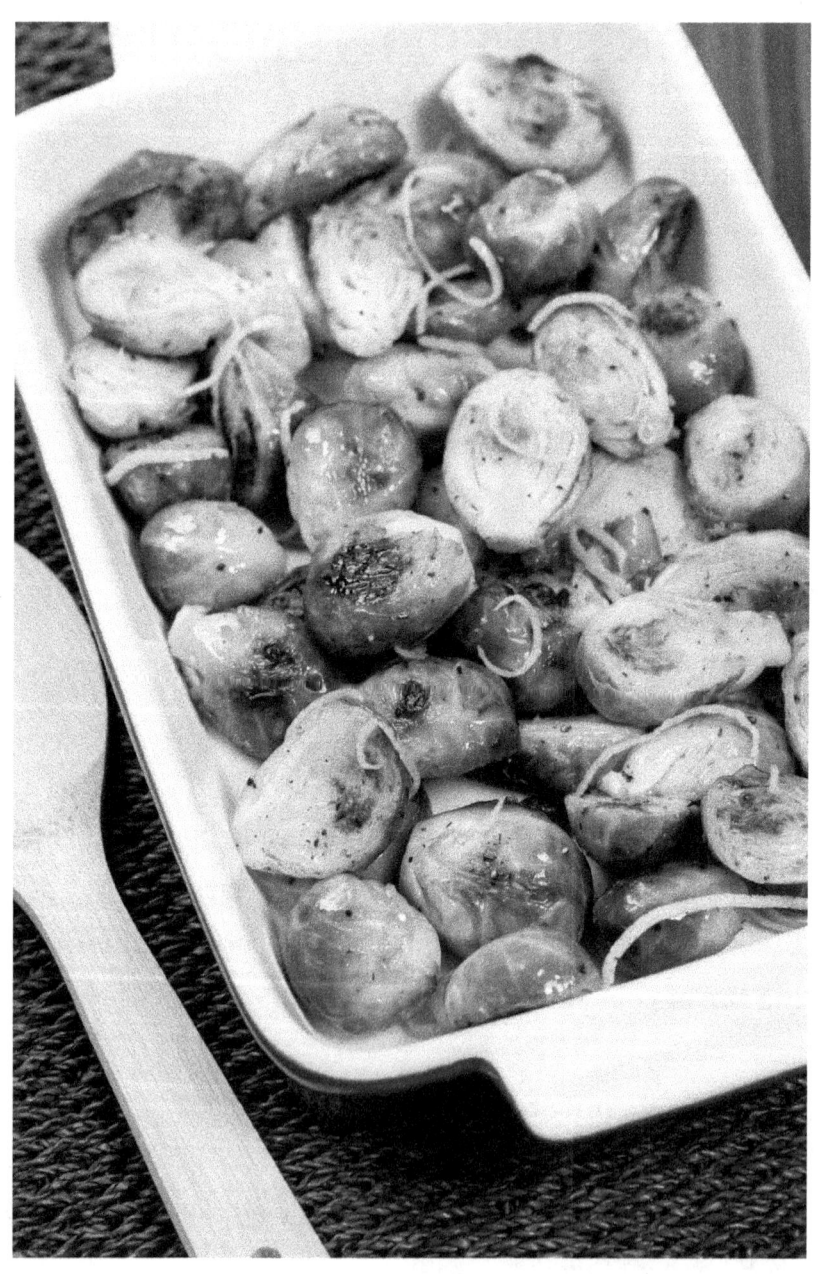

SIMPLE VEGAN BOK CHOY SOUP

Ingredients

- 2 chopped bok choy stalks
- 1 cup vegetable broth
- 1 tsp nutritional yeast
- 2 dashes of garlic powder
- 2 pinches of onion powder
- salt and pepper to taste

Instructions

1. Mix all ingredients in a bowl and mix.
2. Microwave for 3 min

Prep time: 1 min; **Servings:** 1

Macros: Sodium 205 mg Carbs 4 g Fiber 1 g Sugar 2 g

BAKED TOFU FRIES

Ingredients

- 15.5 g of extra tofu firmly drained and squeezed
- 2 Tbsp olive oil
- ½ tsp basil
- ½ tsp oregano
- ¼ tsp pepper
- ¼ tsp cayenne pepper
- ¼ tsp onion powder
- ¼ tsp garlic powder
- Salt and pepper

Instructions

1. Preheat the oven to 375° F.
2. Mix the olive oil and all the herbs and spices.
3. Cut tofu into long strips about ¼ - ½ "thick and cover with marinade.
4. Place the strips on parchment paper and cook for 20 min. Turn and bake another 15-20 min, or until crispy on the outside.

Prep time: 30 min; **Servings:** 4

Macros: Cal 132 | Carbs 3g | Protein 7g | Fat 10 g Saturated Fat 1 g | Cholesterol 0 mg | Sodium 40 mg Potassium 213 mg | Fiber 0 g | Sugar 1 g | Vitamin A: 115 IU | Calcium: 39 mg | Iron: 1.2 mg

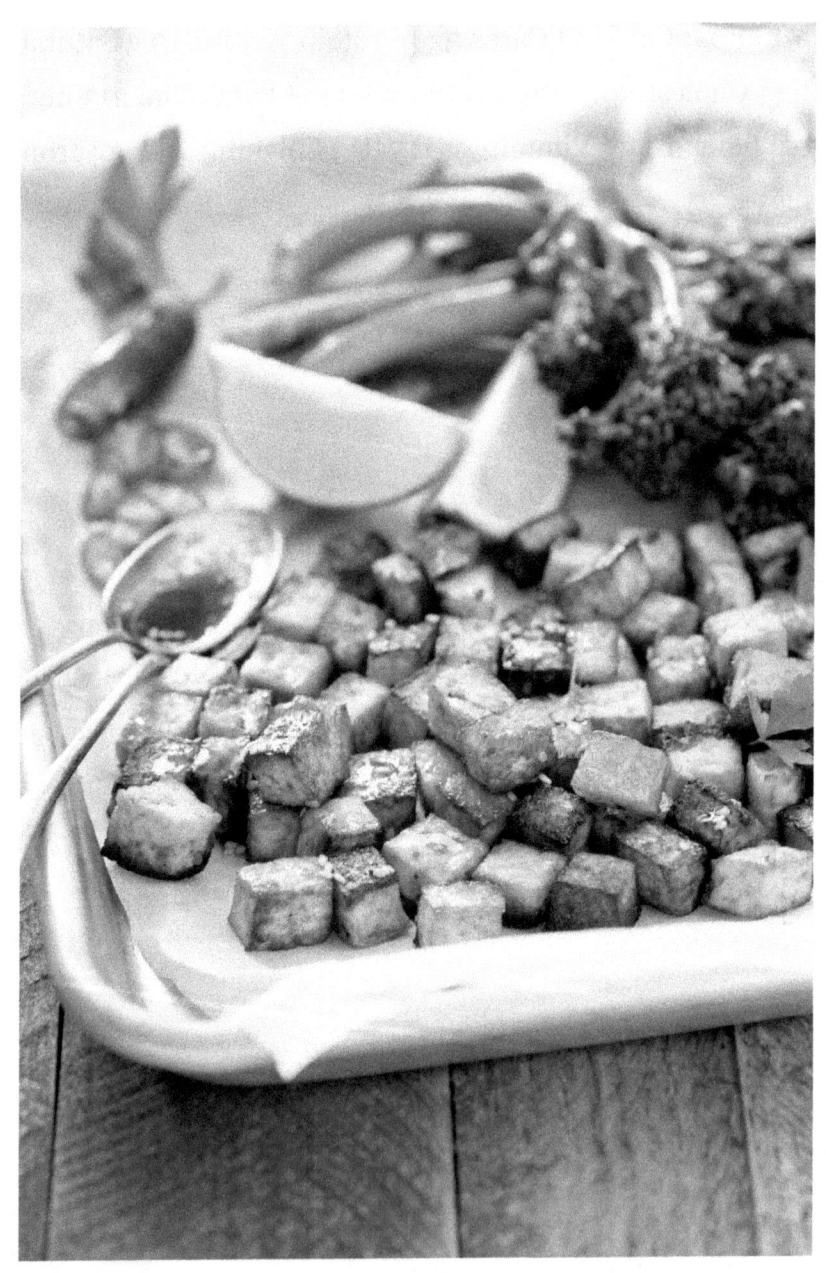

CAULIFLOWER MUSHROOM RISOTTO

Ingredients

- 1 cup medium cauliflower gold 4-5 cups pre-cooked fresh gold frozen cauliflower
- 1 Tbsp ghee or coconut oil
- 1 small onion, diced
- 1 lb of small shiitake mushrooms, sliced or cremini or white mushrooms
- 3 cloves of garlic, finely chopped
- 2 Tbsp coconut amino acids
- 1 cup whole coconut milk
- 1 cup bone broth gold chicken broth gold vegetable broth
- ¼ cup nutritional yeast
- ½ tsp sea salt, to taste
- 2 Tbsp tapioca starch
- Ground black pepper to taste
- Chopped parsley to garnish

Instructions

1. Remove the cauliflower leaves and cut the flowers off the roots.
2. Use a cheese grater or food processor with a rasp accessory and grate the cauliflower to the size of the rice.
3. Add the butter or coconut oil in the instant saucepan and set it to "Sautéed." Cool for 5 min and cover the bottom of the pan.

4. Add the onion, mushrooms and garlic and cook, stirring, for 7 min, until the mushrooms are sweaty and soft.

5. Add the coconut amino acids and sauté 5 min until the vegetables are brown. Turn off the instant pot.

6. Add the cauliflower rice, coconut milk, bone broth, nutritional yeast, and sea salt. Stir together.

7. Close the lid, make sure the valve is closed and set the instant pot to "Manual" for 2 min

8. Release the pressure valve and open the lid.

9. Sprinkle tapioca starch on risotto and stir until thickened. Add more salt if you wish. Add ground black pepper if you use it.

10. Sprinkle with chopped parsley.

Prep time: 5 min; **Servings:** 4

Macros: Cal 299.05 Fat 19.15g Saturated Fat 15.12g Cholesterol 9.6mg Sodium 546.4mg Potassium 1036.52mg Carbs 27.61g Fiber 8.31g Sugar 8.64g Protein 10.62g

SILKY VEGAN CAULIFLOWER SOUP

Ingredients

- 1 small cauliflower gold ½ large cauliflower about 500 g gold 1 lb
- 1 Tbsp olive oil
- 2 cloves of garlic, finely chopped
- 2 sprigs of thyme
- 350 ml or 1 ½ cups of vegetable broth or water
- 120 ml or ½ cups of light coconut milk
- salt and freshly ground black pepper to taste
- 4 Tbsp pomegranate seeds to decorate
- 2 sprigs of thyme to decorate

Instructions

1. Divide the head of cauliflower into florets or cut it more or less. You can use the leaves if you want, but these will change the color of the soup.
2. Fry the chopped garlic in olive oil in a large frying pan until fragrant, about 2 min Add vegetable stock or water, sprigs of thyme and cauliflower flowers. Bring to the boil, cover, reduce heat, and cook for 15-20 min, until the cauliflower is beautiful and!
3. Discard the thyme and mix until smooth with a hand blender or food processor. You may want to work in batches.

4. Add light coconut milk and season with salt and freshly ground black pepper. Garnish with pomegranate seeds and fresh thyme.

Prep time: 10 min; **Servings:** 2

Macros: Cal 184 | Carbs 17 g | Protein 3g | Fat 11 g Saturated Fat 5 g | Sodium 791 mg | Potassium 466 mg Fiber 3g | Sugar 8 g | Vitamin A: 420 IU | Vitamin C: 69.5 mg | Calcium: 35 mg | Iron: 0.7 mg

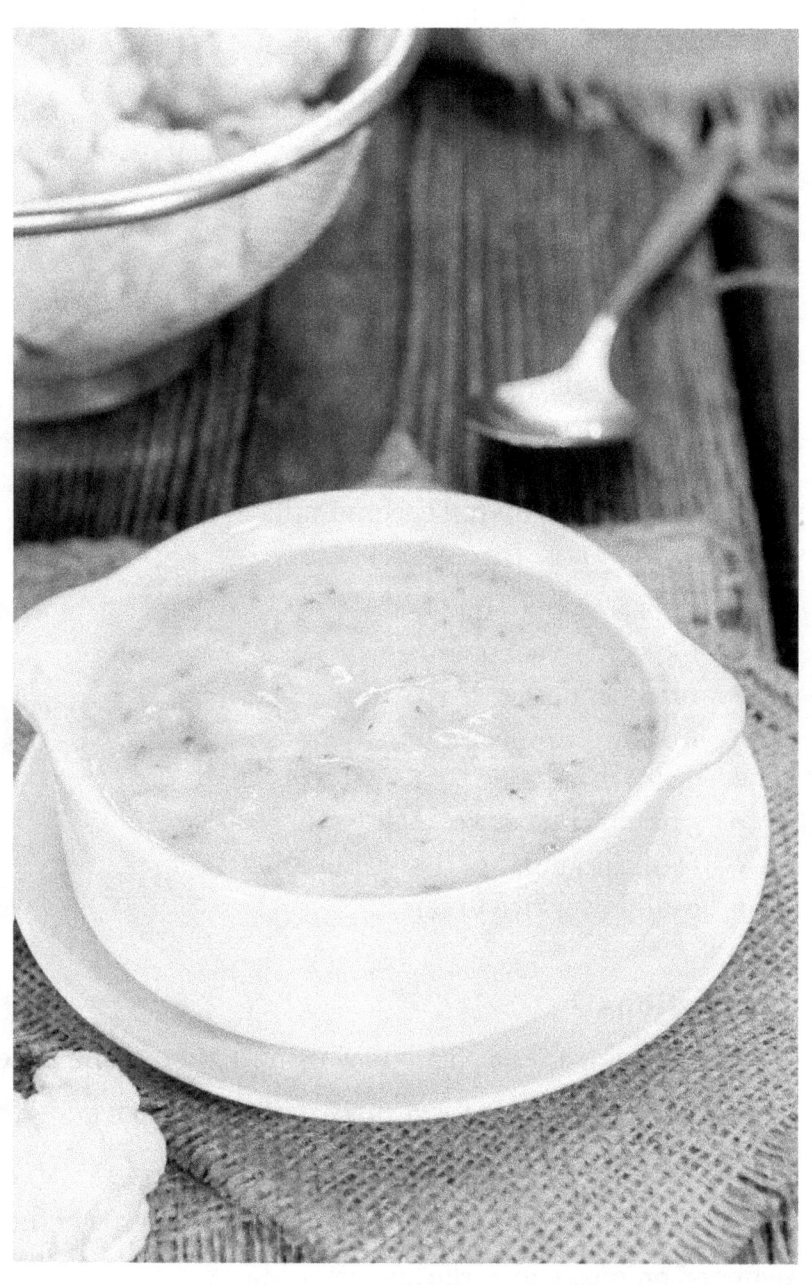

VEGETARIAN RED CURRY STIR FRY

Ingredients

Sauce:
- 1 inch (2.5 cm) fresh ginger
- ½ tsp cumin
- ½ tsp coriander
- 2 Tbsp + 2 tsp red curry paste
- 1 cup or 235 ml full coconut milk

Baked:
- 1 Tbsp coconut oil
- 1 lb gold sweet potatoes
- 1 red pepper
- 1 medium sweet onion
- 2 cloves of garlic
- 5 oz sugar peas
- fresh coriander to decorate
- cauliflower rice to serve

Instructions

1. Grate the ginger in a small bowl using a Microplane zester. Add cumin, cilantro, and red curry paste. Stir, then add coconut and beat until well combined. Put aside.

2. Peel the sweet potatoes and cut into large cubes. Cut the peppers, onions, and garlic and set aside.

3. Heat coconut oil in a large wok or deep pan over medium heat. Add sweet potatoes to the pan and stir to cover. Bake until soft, about 8-10 min.

4. Reduce the heat to medium and add the diced bell pepper and onion to the pan. Cook for another 5 min, stirring regularly.

5. Put the peas and garlic in the pan. Bake for another 3-5 min with continuous stirring until they are sweet and crispy.

6. Remove the pan from the heat and pour the sauce into the pan. Mix to cover the vegetables, extinguish the pan with the sauce. Wait 2-3 min for the sauce to thicken and then serve cauliflower rice (see previous comments)! Top with chopped fresh coriander.

Prep time: 10 min; **Servings:** 4

Macros: Cal 88 Carbs 14g Fat 4g Protein 3g

CREAMY CAULIFLOWER GARLIC RICE

Ingredients

- 6 to 8 cups of chopped cauliflower
- 4 cups vegetable broth + 2 cups water
- ½ cup milk
- 1 ½ cups brown rice
- 1 tsp salt (and more to taste!)
- 2 tsp
- 6-8 cloves minced garlic
- ½ cup cheese mozzarella to cover (more to taste)

Instructions

1. Cook the rice according to the instructions on the package. Put aside.
2. Cook the vegetable broth and water in a large saucepan. Add the cauliflower and cook for about 10 min, until tender. Transfer the cauliflower pieces to a blender or food processor.
3. Puree cauliflower, add extra milk or vegetable broth to a smooth, creamy consistency. Season with salt. For over cooked rice and stir to combine.
4. In a large nonstick skillet, melt butter and add garlic, and cook on low heat

until very fragrant for about 3 to 5 min Add the creamy rice mixture and stir until the butter and garlic are absorbed. Add cheese or mix all the ice to melt. Season with additional salt and pepper.

Servings: 6; **Prep time:** 15 min

Macros: Cal 190 Carbs 23g Fat 9g Protein 5g

HEALTHY CAULIFLOWER FRIED RICE

Ingredients

- 1 chopped cauliflower in florets
- 1 small yellow onion, finely chopped
- ½ cup frozen peas
- ½ cup carrots, diced
- 2 beaten eggs
- 1 Tbsp sesame oil
- ¼ cup low sodium soy sauce
- 1 Tbsp light brown sugar
- ⅛ tsp ground ginger
- 1 pinch of red pepper flakes
- 2 Tbsp chopped green onion

Instructions

1. Chop the cauliflower head into florets and place in a food processor. Press until it starts to look like rice; put aside.
2. A large wok (or skillet) over medium heat and sprinkle with sesame oil. Add the onion, peas, and carrots and cook until tender, about 2 min
3. Meanwhile, mix soy sauce, brown sugar, ginger, and red pepper flakes in a small bowl; set aside.

4. Move the vegetable mixture to the side of the wok and add the beaten egg, stir until they are thoroughly cooked, then add them to the vegetables.

5. Add the cauliflower "rice" and over the soy sauce, mix well. Cook for another 3 to 4 min until cauliflower is tender and soft.

6. Top with green onions.

Prep time: 10 min; **Servings:** 4

Macros: Cal 131 Fat 6.3 g Saturated Fat 1.3 g Carbs 13.5 g Fiber 3 g Protein 6.5 g Sugar 7.1 g

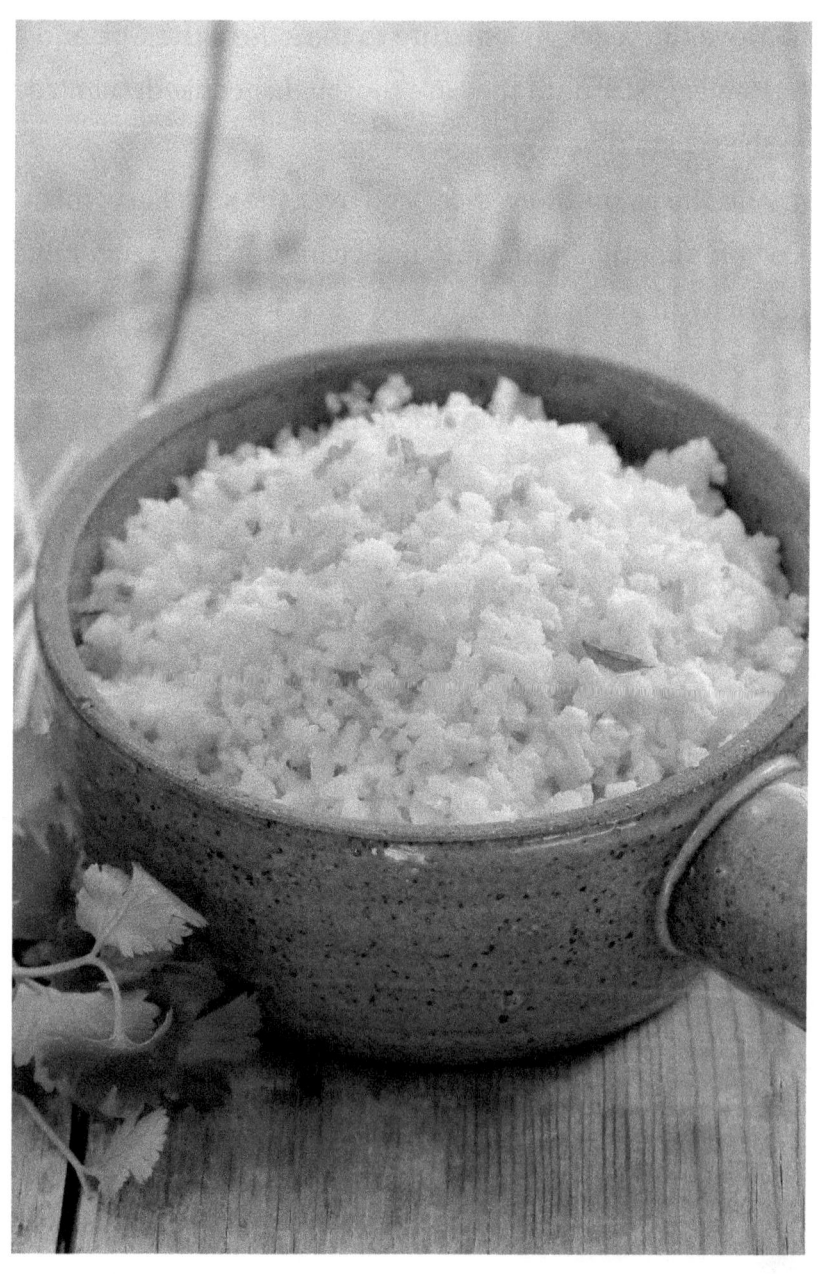

MEXICAN CAULIFLOWER RICE BURRITO BOWL

Ingredients

- 3-3 ½ cups of cauliflower rice
- 1 Tbsp olive oil
- ½ chopped red onion
- 2 garlic cloves, finely chopped
- ½ tsp garlic powder
- 1 tsp cumin
- ½ tsp oregano
- pinch of cayenne pepper
- salt and pepper to taste
- 1 can of black beans 11-14 oz
- 1 diced tomato
- Sliced avocado
- Slices of lemons
- handful of coriander

Instructions

For cauliflower rice:

1. Break the cauliflower into florets and place it in a food processor.
2. The cauliflower pulse is similar to rice. Remove and place on a clean towel or paper towels and wring out any excess liquid.

3. Meanwhile, heat oil over medium heat and add onion and garlic. Saute 2 to 3 min until fragrant and transparent.

4. Add cauliflower, garlic powder, cumin, oregano, cayenne pepper and salt and pepper to taste.

5. Continue cooking regularly, stir for another 8 to 10 min

Bowl assembly:

1. Add Mexican cauliflower
2. black beans, drained and rinsed
3. chopped tomato and chopped red onion remaining
4. slices of avocado
5. sprinkle with lime juice

Prep time: 10 min **Servings:** 2-3

CAULIFLOWER FIESTA RICE SALAD

Ingredients

Salad:

- 1 small cauliflower
- ¼ cup finely chopped red onion
- 1 cup corn
- ½ cup black beans
- 3 jalapeños, finely chopped, without seeds or ribs
- 1 packet (10 g) of tomatoes, grapes or cherries, cut in half
- ⅓ cup fresh cheese or cheese cotija (feta also works)
- ⅓ cup chopped fresh coriander

Dressing:

- 2 lime juice
- 1 orange juice
- 1 Tbsp olive oil
- ½ tsp chili powder
- ¼ tsp cumin
- 1 small clove of garlic

Instructions

1. Prepare the cauliflower rice: cut the cauliflower into large florets. Place the ⅓ of the florets in a food processor. Press until the cauliflower looks like grains of rice. Place the cauliflower rice in a large bowl. Repeat this process 2 more times with the florets.

2. Prepare the salad: add the onion, corn, black beans, jalapeno, tomatoes, cheese, and coriander to the cauliflower rice bowl.

3. Prepare the vinaigrette: add all the ingredients of the vinaigrette to the food processor or blender. Mix until smooth. For salad dressing over salad and mix to combine.

Prep time: 20 min; **Servings:** 8

Macros: Cal 284 Fat 25.6 g Carbohydrate 8.8 g Fiber 3.6 g Sugar 2.2 g Protein 5.8 g Net Carbohydrate 5 g

CURRIED CAULIFLOWER RICE KALE SOUP

Ingredients

- 5-6 cups of cauliflower flowers
- 2 to 3 Tbsp curry powder or curry powder
- 1 tsp garlic powder
- ½ tsp cumin
- ½ tsp sweet pepper
- ¼ tsp sea salt
- 2-3 Tbsp olive oil for frying
- 3/4 cup chopped red onion
- 1 tsp minced garlic
- 2 tsp olive oil or avocado
- 8 kale leaves with the stems removed and chopped
- 2 cups (5 oz) chopped carrots
- 4 cups broth
- 1 cup almond milk or coconut milk
- ½ tsp red gold pepper chili flakes
- ½ tsp black pepper
- Salt after cooking

Instructions

1. Preheat the oven to 400° F.

2. Mix the cauliflower flowers in a small bowl with curry powder, garlic powder, cumin, pepper, salt, and 3 Tbsp oil.

3. Spread cauliflower flowers in a baking dish or on a roasting pan. Place in the oven and cook for 20 to 22 min, but without boiling. Something not cooked.

4. While the cauliflower cools, prepare the remaining vegetables on a chopping board.

5. Then place the bouquets of cauliflower in a food processor or press several times until cauliflower is chopped or "chopped." See the picture in the publication.

6. Once in a while, prepare your pot.

7. Place the onion, 2 tsp oil, and chopped garlic in a large saucepan. Bake for 5 min until fragrant.

8. Then add broth, milk, vegetables, cauliflower "rice" and red pepper and black pepper.

9. Bring it to a boil (make sure the milk does not overheat) and simmer another 20 min until the vegetables are well cooked.

10. If necessary, add a pinch of sea salt when ready to serve.

11. Garnish with herbs and crumble the nuts/cookies with the seeds.

Prep time: 30 min; **Servings:** 4

Macros: Cal 162 Sugar 6 g Sodium 250 mg Fat 8 g Saturated Fat 1.3 g Carbs 20 g Fiber 9 g Protein 6 g

PESTO CAULIFLOWER RICE

Ingredients

- 3 cups of cauliflower rice (see note)
- 1 Tbsp olive oil
- 2 cups shredded kale stalks
- ⅓ to ½ cup extra virgin olive oil
- 1 clove of garlic
- ½ lemon juice
- ⅓ cup grated Parmesan cheese
- 3 Tbsp chopped walnuts

Instructions

1. Add the oil in a large skillet and bring to medium heat. Add the cauliflower and cook until tender.
2. Add pesto ingredients to a food processor to make pesto. Press for a few min until it reaches a thick sauce consistency. The pesto will be ready to be very thick, but it will be a few min later. If it does not decompose, add a little more olive oil until it decomposes. Test and adjust if necessary. Depending on the type of cabbage and your personal preferences, you may want to add cheese, oil, lemon, etc.
3. Add the cauliflower rice pesto. Start with a few Tbsp and add if necessary until you have the desired taste. You may not need the full amount, and you can not use the pesto for another .

4. Serve hot cauliflower rice. Garnish with more Parmesan if desired.

Prep time: 10 min; **Servings:** 4

Macros: Cal 293 Fat 26.6 g Carbohydrate 8.8 g Fiber 3.6 g Sugar 2.2 g Protein 5.8 g Net Carbohydrate 5 g

BLISSFUL BASIL SWEET POTATOES

Ingredients

For roasted sweet potatoes:

- 4 cups sweet potatoes, peeled and cut into 1-inch cubes
- 2 Tbsp grapeseed oil or other heat-tolerant oil
- 1 Tbsp ground cinnamon
- 1 Tbsp smoked pepper
- fine-grained sea salt

For the spicy cauliflower rice

- 1 head of about 6 heartless cups of cauliflower and cut into bouquets 13. 1 Tbsp sesame oil
- 5 onions, sliced and thinly sliced
- 1 cup cherry tomatoes or grapes in wedges
- 2-3 Tbsp apple cider vinegar or rice vinegar
- 1-2 Tbsp reduced-sodium Tamari *
- 1-2 Tbsp garlic and chili paste or Sriracha
- Cup chopped chives
- ¼ cup chopped fresh cilantro

For the smashed avocado

- 1 ripe avocado cut in half, pitted and peeled
- 1 Tbsp fresh lime juice 1 garlic clove, chopped to taste
- Sea salt to taste

Instructions

For roasted sweet potatoes:

1. Preheat the oven to 425 ° F. Cover a large baking sheet with parchment paper.
2. Place the sweet potatoes on a baking sheet, sprinkle with oil, and sprinkle with cinnamon, pepper, and sea salt to taste. Mix to cover.
3. Roast for 25 to 30 min or until soft and return every 15 min
4. For the spicy cauliflower rice
5. Add the cauliflower florets to the bowl of a food processor equipped with an S knife. Press to finely chop the size of the rice kernels.
6. Heat the sesame oil in a large wok gold fry over medium heat. Add the cauliflower, chives, and tomatoes and cook for 8 to 10 min or until the cauliflower softens, stirring occasionally.
7. Mix apple cider vinegar, tamari, and chili and garlic paste in a small bowl. For the sauce over the cauliflower and cook for another 6 to 8 min, or until the "rice" turns into light golden color and the liquid is absorbed, stirring regularly.

Remove from heat and add the onions and cilantro.

For the smashed avocado:

1. Use the back of a fork in a small bowl to mix the avocado, juice lime, garlic, and sea salt.
2. Place the sweet potatoes and cauliflower in bowls, squeeze them together, cover with a generous spoonful of mashed avocado.

Prep time: 15 min; **Servings:** 3

Macros: Cal 605 | Carbs 100 g | Protein 13 g | Fat 22 g | Fiber: 23 g | Sugar 22 g |

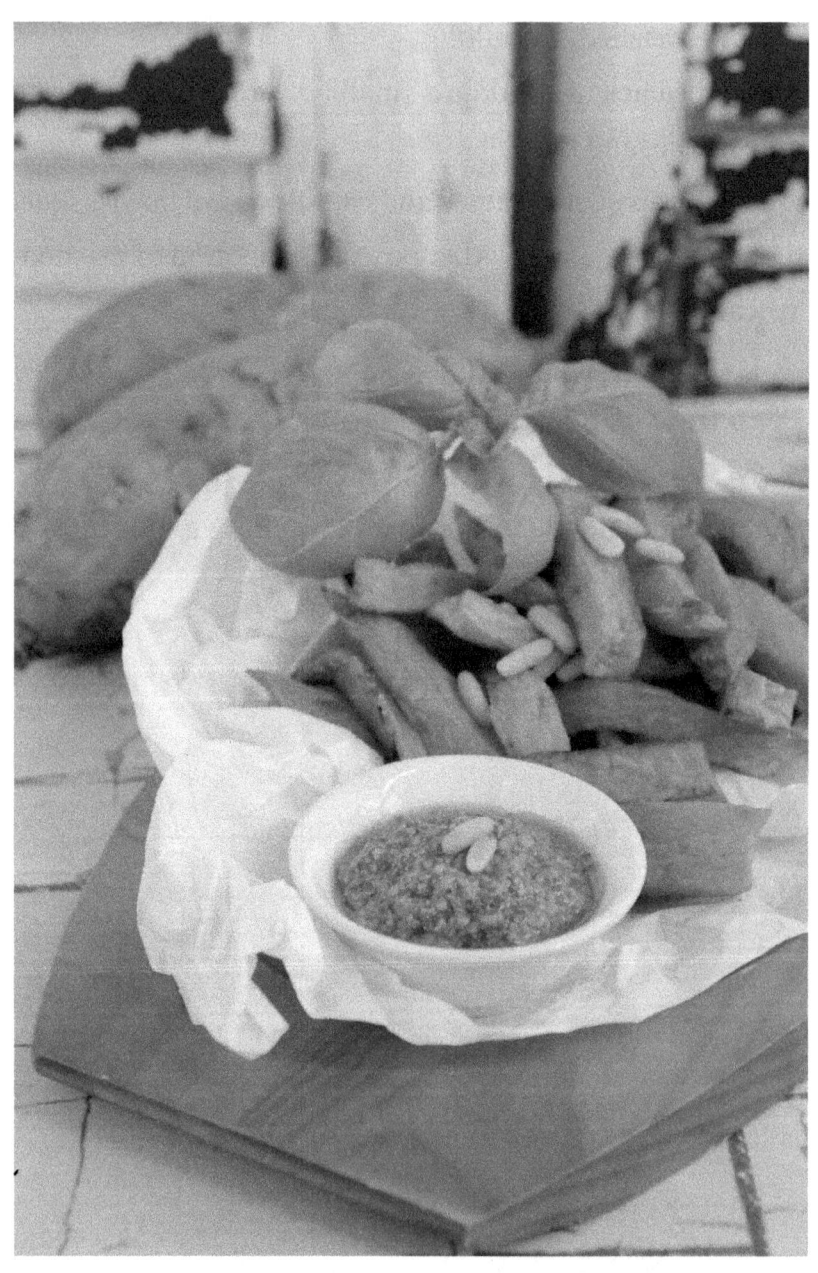

SUSHI VEGAN CAULIFLOWER RICE

Ingredients

- 4 sheets of nori
- 2 cups of cauliflower rice
- 1 red pepper sliced thinly
- 1 avocado, peeled and sliced
- 1 cup finely sliced red cabbage
- 2 green onions sliced all over
- 2 cups of chopped field vegetables
- Peanut sauce
- ¼ cup peanut butter
- 1 tsp stevia
- 2 tsp tamari or Bragg
- 1 tsp Sriracha according to your heat preference
- 2 tsp chopped peanuts to cover

Instructions

1. Place a sheet of nori on a bamboo roll. Cover half a thin layer of cauliflower rice. With thin slices of red pepper, avocado slices, sliced red cabbage, green onion slices, and some field vegetables.
2. Use the bamboo roll with your finger. Roll it firmly to the end.
3. Prepare the sauce by combining peanut butter, agave, Bragg (or tamari), and sriracha. Stir to combine. Add 1 to 3 tsp water to obtain good immersion. Sprinkle top with chopped peanuts.

4. Cut the roll into 5 to 6 cm.

Prep time: 10 min; **Servings:** 8

Macros: Cal 73, Carbs 14g, Fat 5g Protein 9g

SPANISH CAULIFLOWER RICE

Ingredients

- 2 Tbsp avocado oil (or olive oil)
- ½ cup chopped white onion
- 1 lb of cauliflower (about 3 cups)
- 1 cup vegetable broth
- 1 cup enchilada sauce
- garlic salt, chili powder, cumin (optional spices, see comments)
- lime juice (optional)
- coriander (optional, to decorate)

Instructions

1. Heat the oil in a saucepan over high heat. Add chopped onion and stir for 1 minute until it is transparent.

2. Add the curry cauliflower and the vegetable broth. Boil again and stir for a few min

3. Add the sauce enchilada, reduce the heat and cover. Simmer for 15-20 min until most liquids are absorbed.

4. Squeeze the lime juice and the selection of herbs and cover with coriander.

Prep time: 5 min; **Servings:** 4
Macros: Cal 73, Carbs 14g, Fat 5g Protein 9g

FRITTERS WITH CHIPOTLE LIME AIOLI

Ingredients

- 1 cup organic cauliflower without leaves (looking for 4 cups oFresh cauliflower rice)
- 3 large eggs raised in the meadow, a little beaten
- ½ cup blanched almond flour *
- 2 Tbsp coconut flour
- 1 tsp of baking powder (aspect without aluminum and corn)
- 1 tsp garlic powder
- ½ tsp chipotle powder (use chili powder or smoked paprika for less heat or book)
- ½ tsp sea salt (plus sea salt extra flakes to serve)
- freshly ground black pepper
- 2 to 4 Tbsp butter, olive oil, coconut oil, avocado oil or other cooking oil
- ½ cup homemade mayonnaise or avocado oil mayonnaise purchased in store
- ½ tsp chipotle powder
- 1 tsp fresh lime juice
- ½ tsp fresh grated lime
- ⅛ tsp garlic powder

Instructions

1. Remove the green leaves from the head of the cauliflower. Cut the cauliflower head into small florets, remove the kernel and discard. Wash the florets until they are dehydrated. You can also dry with paper towels. You do not want to be wet at all.
2. Add the florets to your food processor. Press several times or process.
3. Put 4 cups of fresh cauliflower rice in a large mixing bowl. Add beaten eggs, almond flour, coconut flour, baking powder, garlic powder, chipotle powder, salt, and pepper. Mix well and let stand for about 10 min. most of the liquid is absorbed, if there is a lot of liquid, it is poured, or a little more coconut flour is added.
4. The heat has a frying pan or skillet. We have a tsp over medium heat. When hot, add enough oil to cover the bottom of the pan. With 2 to 4 Tbsp dough, form burgers with your hands and place them carefully in the hot pan. Work in batches and do not overload the container.
5. Bake until the bottom is brown, about 3 to 4 min, then flip gently and cook for another 3 min Go to a plate with paper towels.
6. Repeat this with the remaining dough and add more if necessary.

7. In a small bowl, mix mayonnaise, chipotle, juice and lemon zest, and garlic powder.

Prep time: 15 min; **Servings:** 4

Macros: Cal 605 | Carbs 100 g | Protein 13 g | Fat 22 g | Fiber: 23 g | Sugar 22 g |

CAULIFLOWER BIBIMBAP

Ingredients

- 1 cup medium cauliflower
- 2 cups of kale
- 1 carrot peeled and cut into matches
- 6 oz sliced shiitake mushrooms
- 1 cup bean sprouts
- 2 cups fresh spinach
- 2 eggs
- 2 Tbsp low sodium soy gold sauce more, to taste
- 2 Tbsp sesame oil or more, to taste
- 2 Tbsp Sriracha sauce to taste
- Salt + pepper
- Sesame seeds (optional)

Instructions

1. For cauliflower rice: cut it into small pieces and place it in a food processor until it looks like grains of rice. For a large bowl, cover with a paper towel and microwave for 4 min
2. The boil has a pan of water. Add the bean springs and the bleach until they are slightly soft. Do not cook it too much.
3. Drain and place in a bowl. Add 1 Tbsp sriracha sauce, 1 tsp sesame oil, and 1 tsp sesame seeds and stir with the bean sprouts. Put aside.
4. Blanch the carrots in the same way and make sure you do not overcook them.

5. Brown the mushrooms in a medium with 1 Tbsp sesame oil until smooth. Add 1 Tbsp soy sauce to the fungus and place it on a plate.

6. Then cook the spinach in the kitchen and add a little soy sauce to season. Set aside spinach

7. Repeat the same process with kale

8. Fry the egg.

9. Stir in a bowl with cauliflower at the bottom, followed by vegetables and top with fried eggs.

Prep time: 15 min; **Servings:** 2

Macros: Cal 306 Fat 19g Saturated Fat 3g Cholesterol 163mg Carbs 23g Fiber 5g Sugar 7g Protein 14g

ROASTED BOK CHOY

Ingredients

- 1 large cup Bok choy
- ¼ cup avocado oil
- 1 tsp sea salt
- ½ tsp black pepper
- 4 cloves of garlic (minced)

Instructions

1. Preheat the oven to 425 F.
2. Cut the bok choy into quarters or eighths.
3. Place the bok choy in a single layer on a large baking sheet. Spray with 2 Tbsp avocado oil. Repeat the oil, salt, and pepper on the other side.
4. Spread chopped garlic through the bok choy with your hands.
5. Roast the bok choy for 10 min in the oven on the lower rack until the leaves begin to lightly char.

Prep time: 10 min; **Servings:** 4

Macros: Cal 152 Fat 14g Protein 3g Total Carbs 5g Net Carbs 3g Fiber 2g Sugar 2g

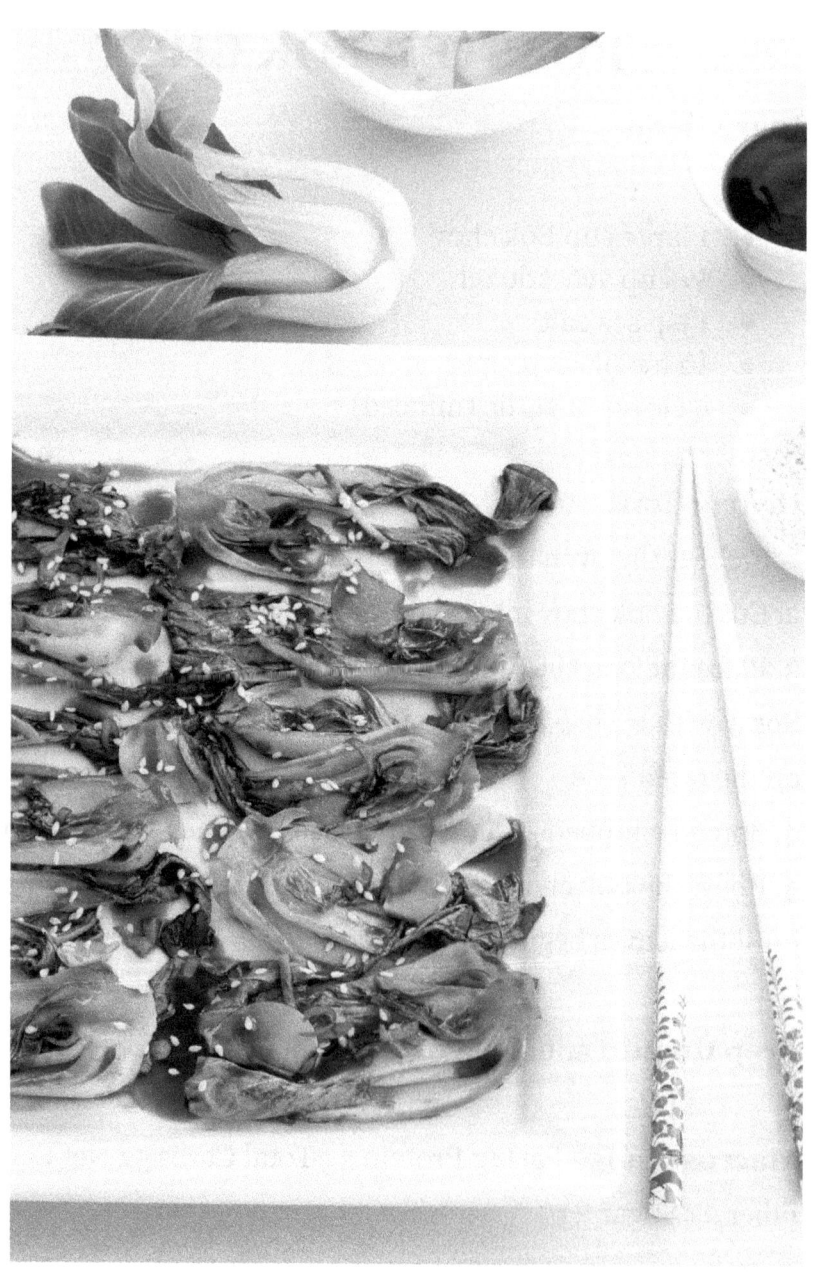

VEGAN SHAKSHUKA

Ingredients

- 2 Tbsp olive oil
- 1 8 g oFirm dry tofu
- 3 tsp harissa
- 1 Tbsp tomato puree
- 2 red bell peppers, cut into small cubes
- 1 tsp smoked pepper
- 1 large onion, diced
- 4 minced teeth
- 1 pinch of salt
- 1 tsp cumin
- 1 pinch of sugar
- 28 g of tomatoes, canned or freshly cut
- 2 tsp Za'atar grilled
- ½ cup labneh without sugar or vegan yogurt

Instructions

1. Cut the tofu in half lengthwise. Dry and cut them into cubes.
2. With olive oil, tomato puree, smoked pepper, harissa, onion, red peppers, garlic, sugar, cumin, and salt. Sauce until peppers are tender for 6-8 min Stir regularly.
3. Add the tomatoes and simmer for ten min until the vegetables. Place each cup or round tofu in the sauce, press the sauce only when it is only visible, and the rest is immersed in the sauce. Let it simmer for ten min.

4. Throw the Za'atar up and serve with plain bread and Labneh.

Prep time: 10 min; **Servings:** 4

Macros: Cal 151, Carbs 15g, Fat 5g Protein 9g

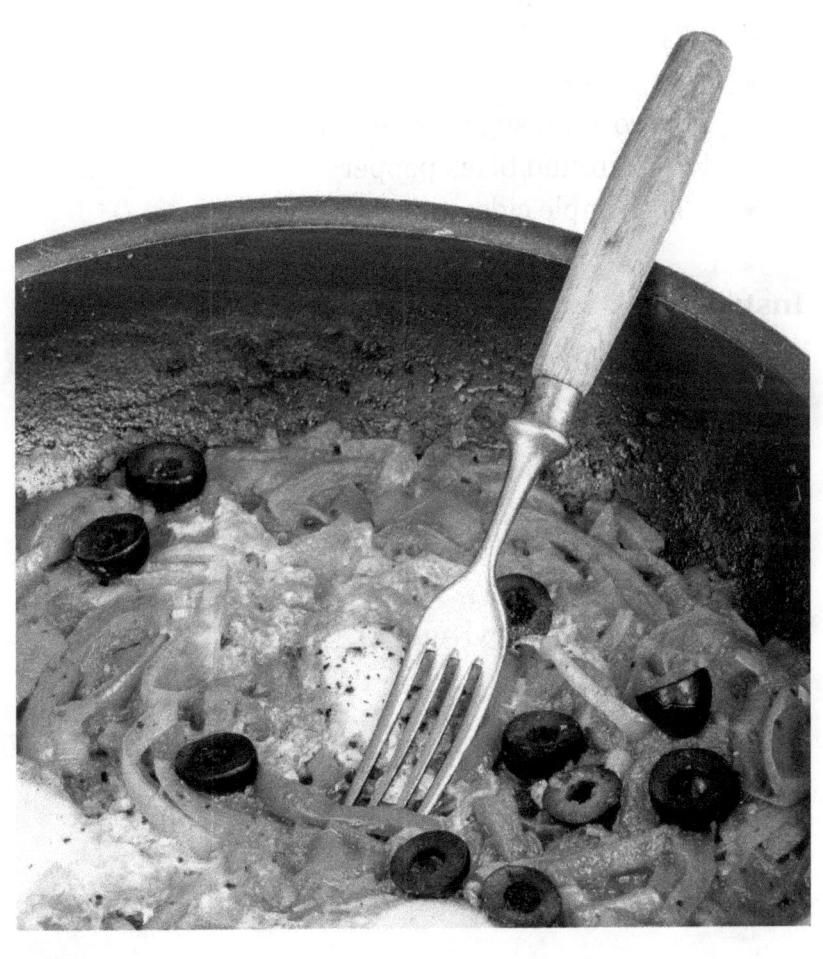

REFRIGERATED VEGETABLE SALAD

Ingredients

- 1 lb of pickles or English cucumbers
- ½ medium onion, thinly sliced
- 2 Tbsp fresh dill packed
- 1 tsp sea salt
- 1 tsp coconut sugar or more to taste
- ¼ tsp ground black pepper
- 2 Tbsp apple cider vinegar

Instructions

1. Use a mandolin or sharp knife to cut the cucumbers into thin slices.
2. Place in a large bowl.
3. Add the remaining ingredients and mix gently.

Prep time: 5 min; **Servings:** 4

Macros: Cal 24 Sodium 586mg Potassium 174 Carbs 4g Fiber 1g Sugar 2g

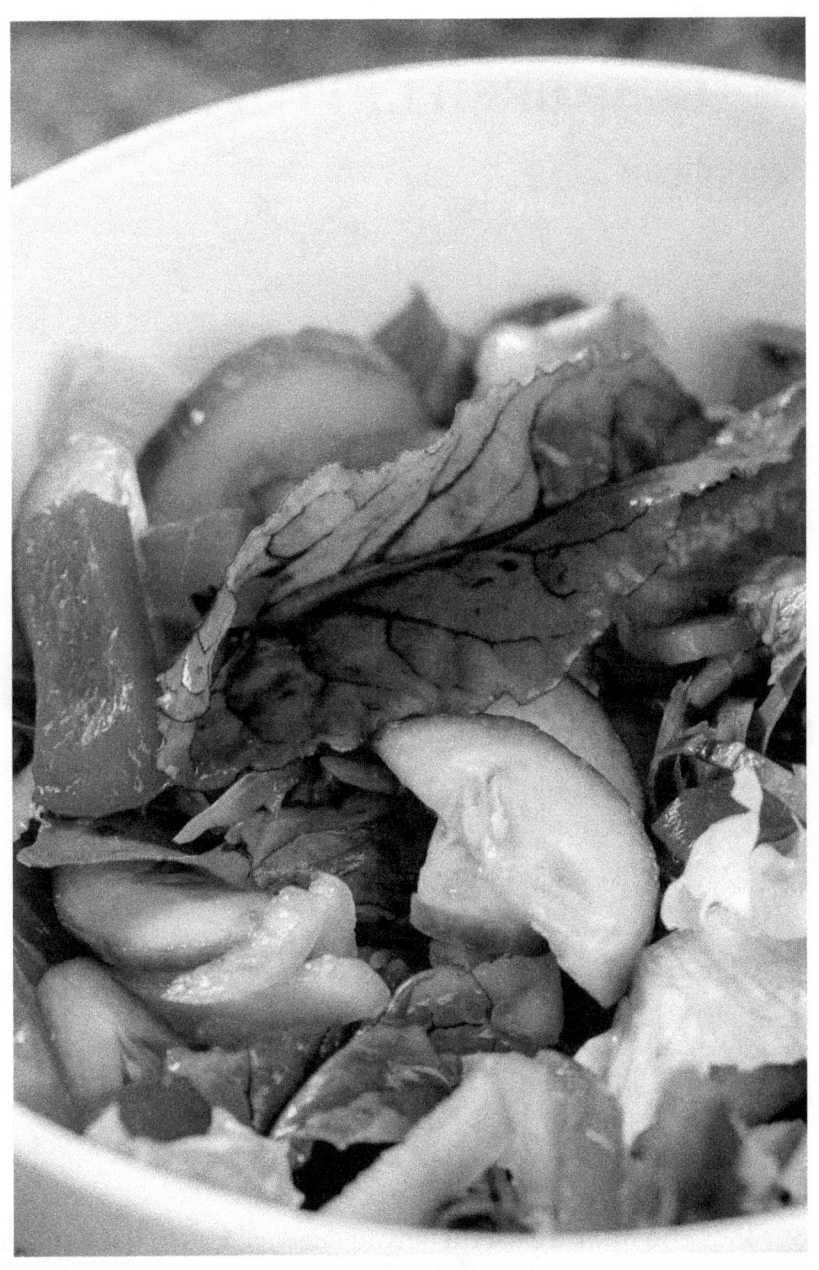

GINGER, SESAME, WALNUT AND HEMP SEED LETTUCE WRAPS

Ingredients

Sauce:

- 2 Tbsp tamari
- 1 Tbsp maple syrup
- 1 tsp roasted sesame oil
- 2 Tbsp brown rice vinegar
- 1 Tbsp chopped ginger

Filling:

- 1 cup chopped walnuts
- ½ cup hemp seeds
- 2 chopped dates
- ½ cup chopped cucumber
- ¼ cup chopped carrots
- optional sesame seeds

Instructions

1. Mix the sauce ingredients.
2. Add chopped walnuts, hemp seeds, dates, cucumber, and carrots. Put in the fridge for at least 1 hour to mix the ingredients.
3. Stack the mixture on the lettuce leaves. Cover with sesame seeds if desired.

Prep time: 10 min; **Servings:** 4

Macros: Cal 382 | Carbs 13 g | Protein 14 g | Fat 31 g | Saturated Fat 2g | Cholesterol 0 mg | Sodium 510 mg | Potassium 230 mg Fiber: 3 g | Sugar 6g | Vitamin A: 1465 IU | Vitamin C: 1.4 mg Calcium: 72 mg | Iron: 4.5 mg

ROASTED PEPPERS AND ONIONS

Ingredients

- 1 red pepper
- 1 orange pepper
- 1 yellow pepper
- 1 small onion
- 1 tsp avocado oil
- ½ tsp smoked pepper
- ¼ tsp oregano
- A pinch of salt
- A pinch of pepper

Instructions

1. Preheat the oven to 400° F.
2. Chop peppers and onions.
3. Place the vegetables in slices on a baking sheet and mix with the oil and herbs.
4. Bake in 1 layer for 20 min
5. Stir after 20 min, then cook another 10 min if necessary.

Prep time: 5 min; **Servings:** 4

Macros: Cal 177 | Carbs 29 g | Protein 4g | Fat 5 g Sodium 15 mg Potassium 856 mg | Fiber 7 g | Sugar 13 g | Vitamin A: 8180°IU | Vitamin C: 527.5 mg | Calcium: 29 mg | Iron: 2 mg

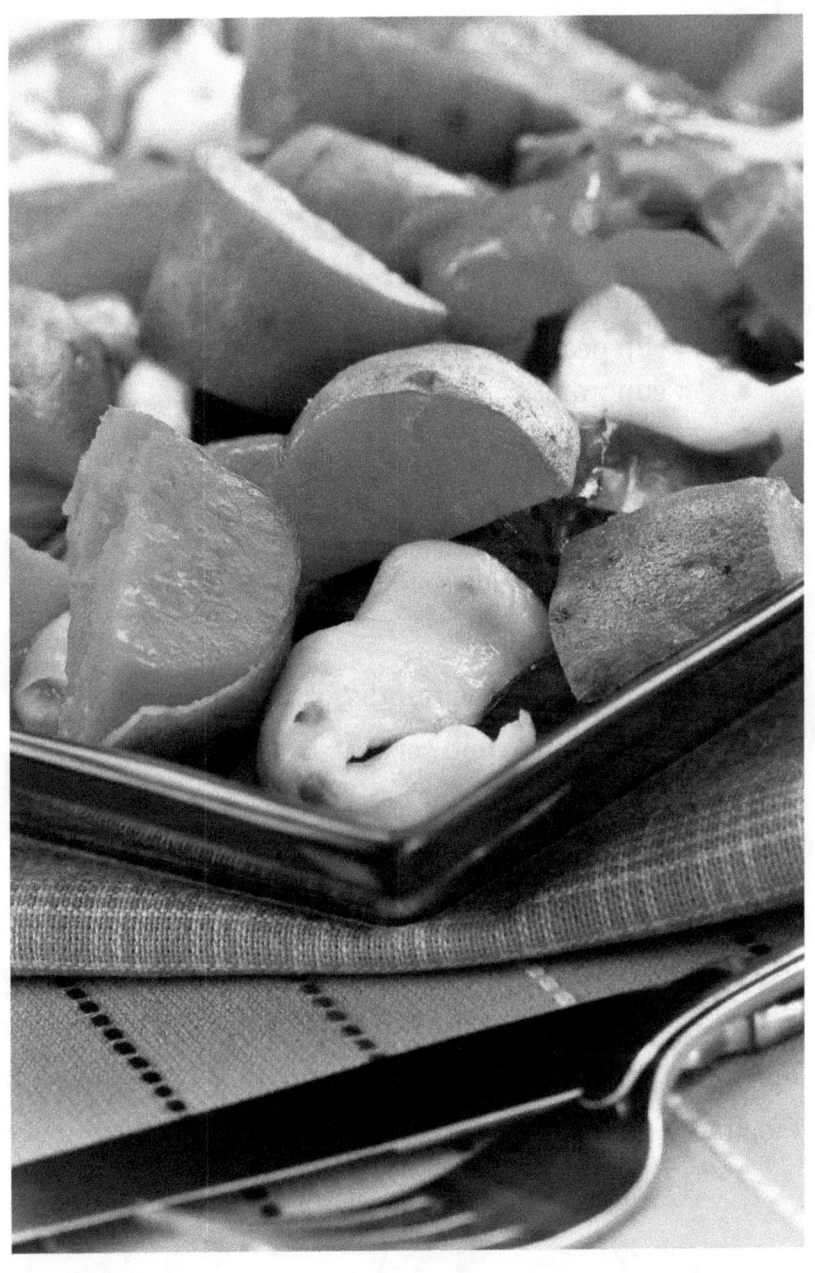

CURRY PUMPKIN SOUP

Ingredients

- 13.5 g of coconut milk
- 15 g of pumpkin puree
- 2 Tbsp Thai red curry paste
- ¼ cup peanut butter
- ¼ cup water
- 2 tsp lime juice

Instructions

1. Put all the ingredients except the lime juice in a saucepan. Bring to a boil and simmer.
2. Boil until the peanut butter dissolves.
3. Add the juiced lime and serve.

Prep time: 5 min; **Servings:** 4

Macros: Cal 328 | Carbs 15 g | Protein 7g | Fat 29 g Saturated Fat 20 g | Cholesterol 0 mg | Sodium 92 mg Potassium 534 mg | Fiber 4 g | Sugar 5g | Vitamin A: 17725 IU | Vitamin C: 6.8 mg | Calcium: 62 mg | Iron: 5.1 mg

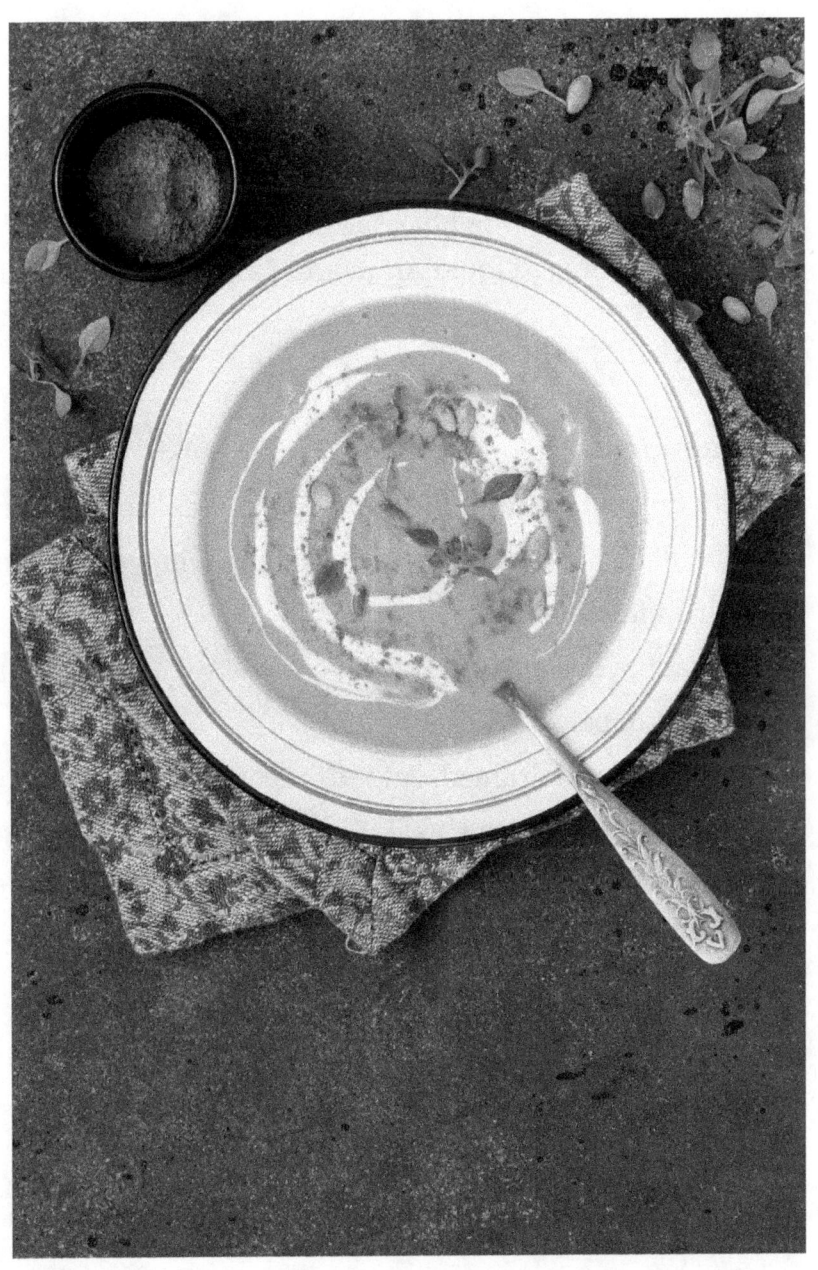

TOFU PERFECT BAKED CRISPY

Ingredients

- 1 extra stable tofu block
- ¼ cup Bragg Liquid Amino Acids Golden Soy or Tamari Sauce
- 1 Tbsp cornflour

Instructions

1. Drain the tofu: remove the tofu from the package and wrap the tofu block with paper towels. Carefully remove the excess moisture and set aside.
2. Preheat the oven to 425 F and cover the baking sheet with parchment paper.
3. Once the tofu is drained, cut into cubes and place in a large bowl. Pour Bragg and sprinkle the cornflour on the tofu and stir gently until it is evenly covered, and the cornstarch is not dry.
4. Place the cubes on a sheet and cook for 25 to 30 min. Flip halfway through.

Prep time: 10 min; **Servings:** 4

Macros: Cal 98 Fat 5 g Saturated fat 1 g Carbs 2 g Protein 12 g

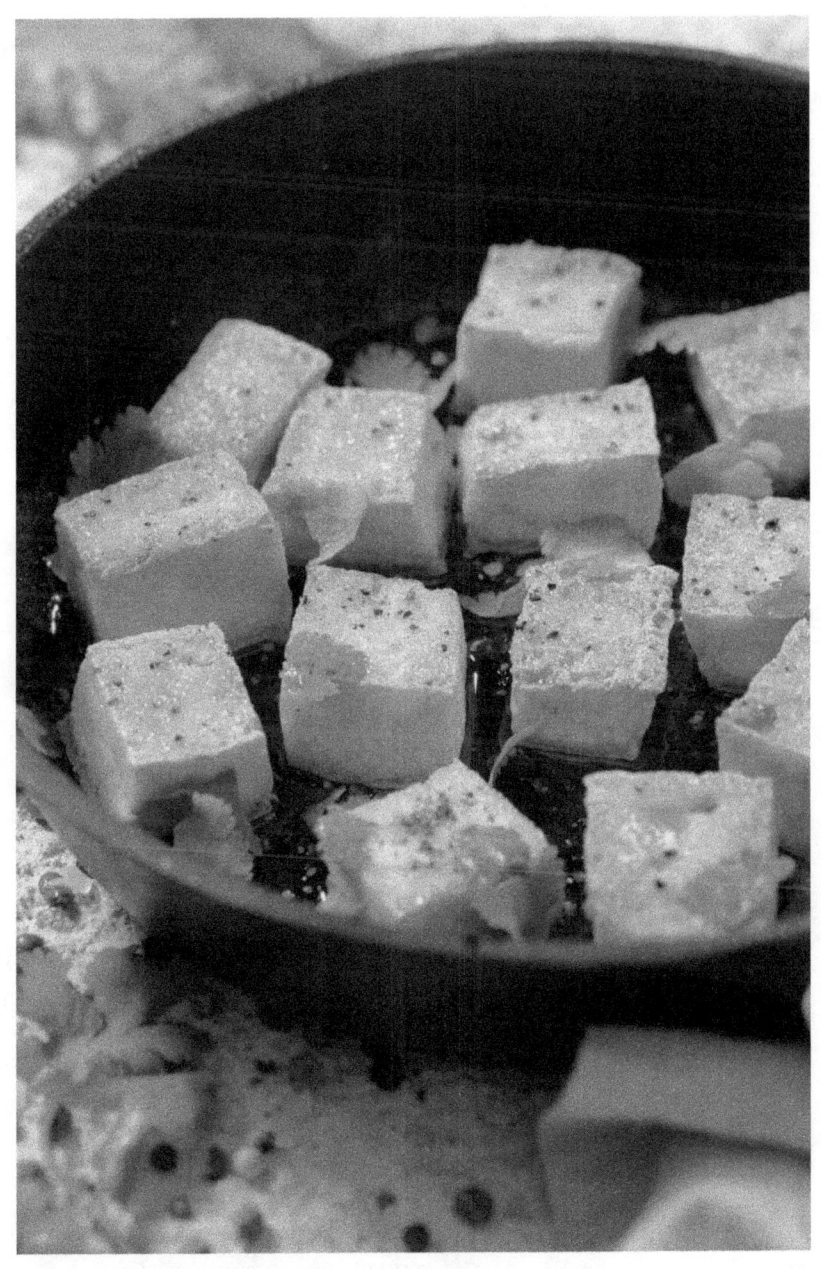

KETO CAULIFLOWER STUFFING

Ingredients

- 1 large cauliflower (cut into small flowers)
- 1 large onion (sliced)
- ¼ cup celery (chopped)
- 2 cloves of garlic (minced)
- ¼ cup olive oil (you can also use butter)
- ½ tsp bird spices
- ½ tsp dried thyme
- ½ tsp ground sage
- 1 tsp sea salt
- ¼ tsp black pepper
- 2 Tbsp fresh parsley
- ¼ cup nuts

Instructions

Preheat the oven to 450° F. Cover the baking sheet with aluminum foil and grease well.

Mix the chopped cauliflower, onions, celery, and garlic in a large bowl. Mix with olive oil, chicken herbs, sage, thyme, sea salt, and black pepper. Spread mixture in a single layer on the baking sheet. Roast in the oven for about 15 min, until the onions are tender and the cauliflower begins to brown. A little.

Add the fresh parsley and nuts in the pan and mix everything. Roast again 10 to 15 min, until the pecans are lightly toasted, the cauliflower is golden brown, and the onions begin to caramelize.

Prep time: 10 min **Servings:** 4

Macros: Cal 95 Fat 7g Protein 2g Total Carbs 7g Net Carbs 4g Fiber 3g Sugar 3

KETO VEGAN PIZZA STICKS

Ingredients

- 1 extra stable tofu block
- ¼ cup + 1 Tbsp tomato sauce
- 2 Tbsp + 2 tsp nutritional yeast
- pinches of dried basil

Instructions

1. Drain the tofu: wrap a block of tofu in a paper towel. Place a cutting board on the tofu block. Press evenly on the top of the block by placing a cookbook on the cutting board. Drain the tofu for about 15-20 min
2. While the tofu is dripping, preheat the oven to 425 and cover the baking sheet with parchment paper.
3. Cut the tofu into 16 thin pieces and place them on a baking sheet.
4. Spread 1 tsp marinara sauce on each pizza bar.
5. Sprinkle ½ tsp nutritional yeast on each bar.
6. Sprinkle with basil on tofu sticks, to taste.

Prep time: 10 min; **Servings:** 4

Macros: Cal 133 Fat 6 g Saturated fat 1 g Sodium 21 mg Potassium 313 mg Carbs 7 g Fiber 3 g Protein 14 g

ZUCCHINI NOODLES WITH AVOCADO SAUCE

Ingredients

- 1 zucchini
- 1 ¼ cup basil (30 g)
- ⅓ cup water (85 ml)
- 4 pine nuts Tbsp
- 2 Tbsp lemon juice
- 1 lawyer
- 12 sliced cherry tomatoes

Instructions

1. Make zucchini noodles with a peeler or a spiralizer.
2. Mix remaining ingredients (except cherry tomatoes) in a blender until smooth.
3. Mix noodles, avocado sauce, and cherry tomatoes in a bowl.

Prep time: 10 min **Servings:** 2

Macros: Cal 313 Sugar 6.5 g Sodium 22 mg Fat 26.8 g saturated Fat 3.1 g Carbs 18.7 g Fiber 9.7 g Protein 6.8 g

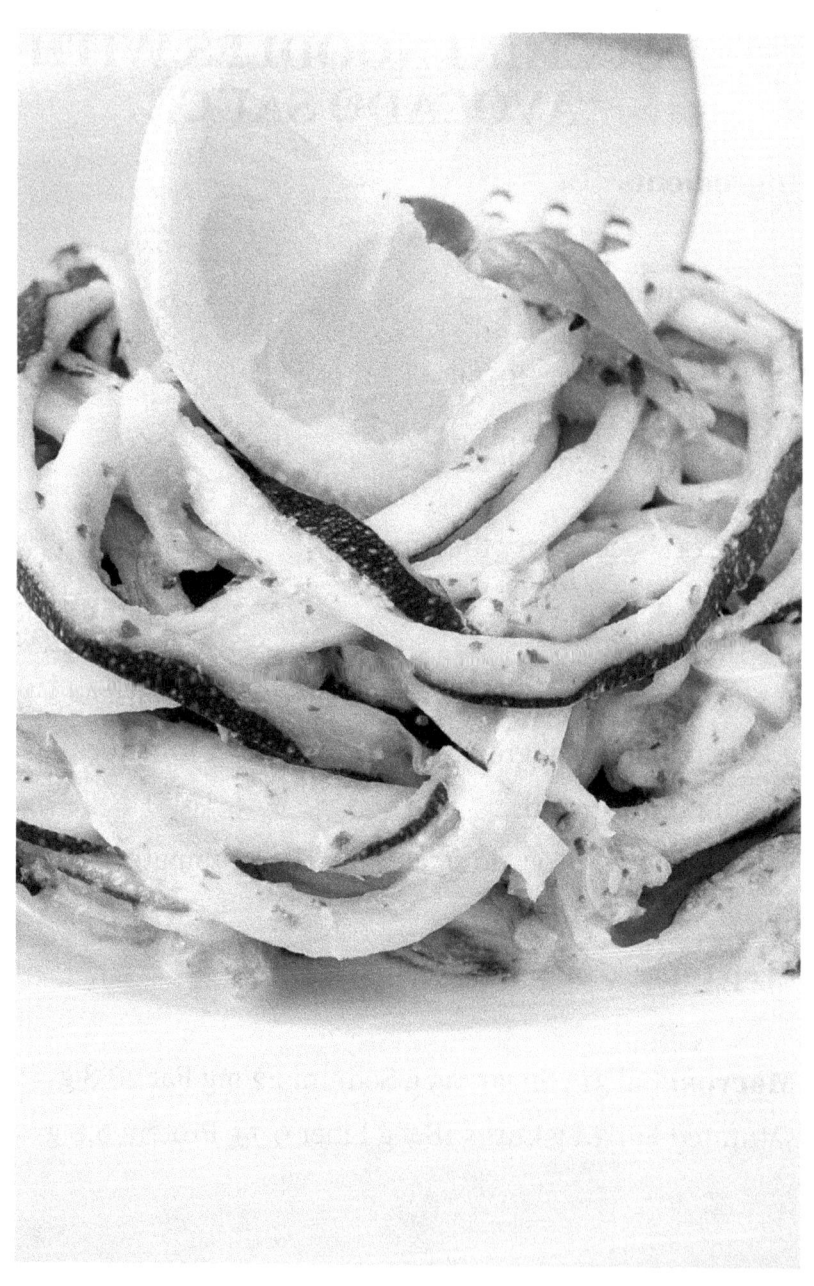

VEGAN TOFU BUFFALO WINGS

Ingredients

- 1 block of extra firm organic tofu from House Foods
- ¼ cup hot sauce of your choice
- 1 Tbsp cornflour
  For an additional coating:
- ½ cup water
- 2 Tbsp hot sauce
- ½ tsp garlic powder
- ¼ tsp onion powder
- ¼ tsp pepper
- salt and pepper to taste
- 4 drops of Monk Fruit liquid Lakanto sweetener gold
- 8 drops of liquid stevia extract
- 1.5 tsp cornflour + 1 Tbsp water

Optional:

- Serve with a Vegan Ranch Vinaigrette

Instructions

1. Cut the drained tofu into 32 pieces of the same size and place in a large mixing bowl.
2. For the hot sauce, sprinkle the cornflour on the tofu and stir gently until it is evenly covered, and the cornstarch is not dry.

3. Heat a nonstick skillet over little heat (or sprinkle a nonstick skillet with an oil spray).

4. Cook the tofu for 3-4 min (until the bottom is golden), turn and cook the other side for another 3 min

5. While baking tofu, preheat the oven to 425F, line a baking sheet with parchment paper and set aside.

6. Beat all additional ingredients in a skillet and heat over medium heat. Let it thicken until it reaches the desired consistency (I did it 3 min), stirring occasionally. Put aside.

7. When the tofu is cooked, put it back in a large mixing bowl, add half the new coating mixture, and stir.

8. Place the tofu on a baking sheet and bake for 10 min on each side.

9. Remove from the oven, cover with an additional coating. And serve with a Vegan Ranch salad dressing if desired.

Prep time: 10 min; **Servings:** 8

Macros: Cal 25 Fat 1 g 2% Sodium 219 mg Potassium 35 mg Carbs 1 g Protein 3 g

CAULIFLOWER RICE PILAF WITH HEMP SEED

Ingredients

- ½ cup cauliflower (2 cups of cauliflower rice)
- ½ cup hemp seeds
- 4 chopped dates
- ½ tsp turmeric
- ½ tsp cumin
- ½ cup low sodium vegetable broth
- ¼ cup sliced almonds
- Salt and pepper

Instructions

1. If you are using a cauliflower head, cut it into large pieces, and place it in the food processor. Mix until it looks like a rice consistency.
2. Chopped dates, turmeric, caraway, vegetable broth, and salt and pepper. Cook until liquid is absorbed, about 5 min
3. Add the sliced almonds.

Prep time: 5 min; **Servings:** 4

Macros: Cal 224 | Carbs 12 g | Protein 12 g | Fat 14 g Saturated Fat 1 g | Cholesterol 0 mg | Sodium 139 mg | Potassium 308 mg Fiber: 3 g | Sugar 6g | Vitamin A: 190 IU | Vitamin C: 34.7 mg | Calcium: 71 mg | Iron: 4.4 mg

GRILLED GARLIC CAULIFLOWER

Ingredients

- 1 medium cauliflower
- ¼ cup avocado oil (or light olive oil)
- ½ tsp sea salt
- ¼ tsp black pepper
- 4 garlic cloves, finely chopped

Instructions

1. Preheat the oven to 400° F. Grease a baking sheet.
2. Cut the cauliflower into ½ inch (1.25 cm) thick slices, then cut into small florets.
3. Mix the cauliflower in a large bowl with oil, salt sea, black pepper, and chopped garlic.
4. Place the cauliflower in a single layer on the baking sheet.
5. Bake for about 15-20 min, or until golden on the bottom. Turn over and cook for another 5 to 10 min.

Prep time: 5 min **Servings:** 4

Macros: Cal161 Fat14g Protein 2g Total Carbs 8g Net Carbs 5g Fiber 3g Sugar 2g

MASHED TURNIPS

Ingredients

- ¼ cup coconut milk or almond milk
- 2 Tbsp coconut oil or butter with butter
- salt and ground black pepper to taste
- chives to decorate
- 1.5 lbs of turnips, peeled and quartered

Instructions

1. Cook the turnips in a saucepan until soft (about 30 to 45 min). Remove from water and place in a large bowl or food processor.
2. Add coconut oil with a taste of butter (or coconut milk) and almond milk (or ghee).
3. Mix with an electric mixer or food processor. Add low-carb milk if necessary. Add salt and pepper to taste.

Prep time: 10 min; **Servings:** 4

Macros: Cal 135 | Carbs 11 g | Protein 1g | Fat 10 g Saturated Fat 8 g | Cholesterol 0 mg | Sodium 115 mg Potassium 355 mg | Fiber 3g | Sugar 6g | Vitamin C: 35.7 mg | Calcium: 54 mg | Iron: 1 mg

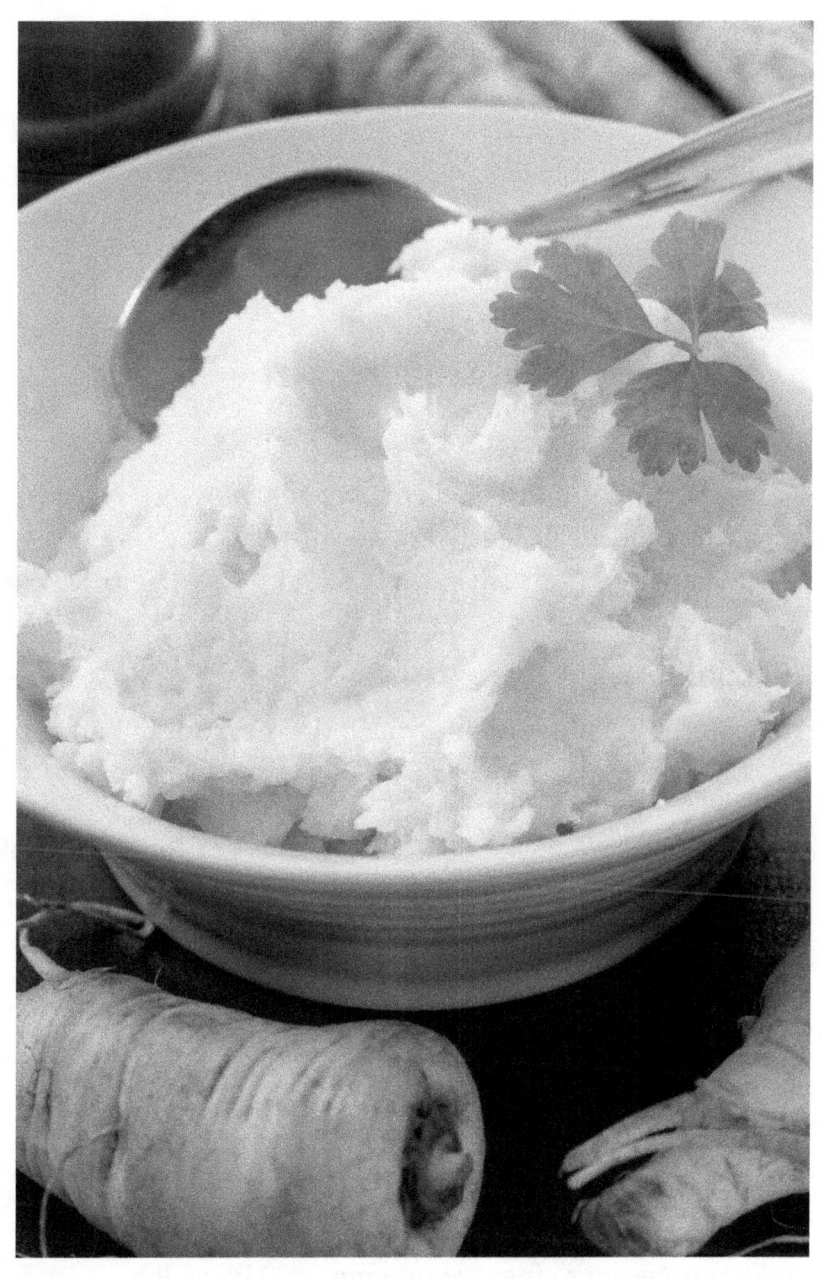

ENSALADA TALONG – FILIPINO EGGPLANT SALAD

Ingredients

- 2 small eggplants
- 2 Tbsp apple cider vinegar
- 1 Tbsp white vinegar
- ½ tsp onion powder
- 1 tsp garlic powder
- salt and ground black pepper to taste
- roasted garlic garnished to garnish
- parsley to garnish

Instructions

1. Wash the eggplants well with cold water. Cut in half to open the eggplant and cut in pieces 1 to 2 centimeters long.
2. Using a baking sheet, place foil, and place the eggplant pieces down with the skin. Season with salt and pepper. Let stand 15 min wrap in aluminum foil.
3. Cook eggplant in an oven preheated to 400° For 10 to 15 min or until smooth. Let cool for 10 to 15 min,
4. After cooling, remove the skin and separate the eggplant into pieces with a fork.
5. Sprinkle onion and garlic powder and mix.
6. For apple cider vinegar and vinegar. Mix well.
7. Put in a bowl and cover with chopped garlic and wansoy.

Prep time: 35 min; **Servings:** 4

Macros: Cal 52 | Carbs 12 g | Protein 2g | Sodium 82 mg | Potassium 415 mg | Fiber 7 g | Sugar 5g | Vitamin A: 100 IU | Vitamin C: 7.4 mg | Calcium: 20 mg Iron: 0.5 mg

KETO MASHED POTATOES

Ingredients

- 1 head of cauliflower (only florets, stems wholly removed)
- 3 cloves garlic (minced)
- 3 Tbsp butter (fixed size, then melted, you can also replace olive oil or ghee without dairy products)
- 1 Tbsp whole coconut milk (or thick cream for paleo)
- 3/4 tsp sea salt (adjust to taste)
- A pinch of black pepper (adjust to liking)
- 1 chopped Tbsp (finely chopped)

Instructions

1. Cook the cauliflower on the hotplate or in the microwave.
2. Stove Method: Boil a pan of water with a Tbsp (14 g) of salt. Add cauliflower and simmer gently (about 5-6 min). Drain well.
3. Microwave Method: Place the cauliflower flowers in a large bowl with 2 Tbsp water. Cover with plastic wrap so that the plastic does not touch the cauliflower. Microwave at high temperature for about 10 min, until they are very soft, Drain well.
4. Meanwhile, put the garlic, melted butter, and milk in a potent food processor or blender.

Prep time: 10 min; **Servings:** 4

Macros: Cal139 Fat10g Protein 4g Total Carbs 12g Net Carbs 7g Fiber5g Sugar5g

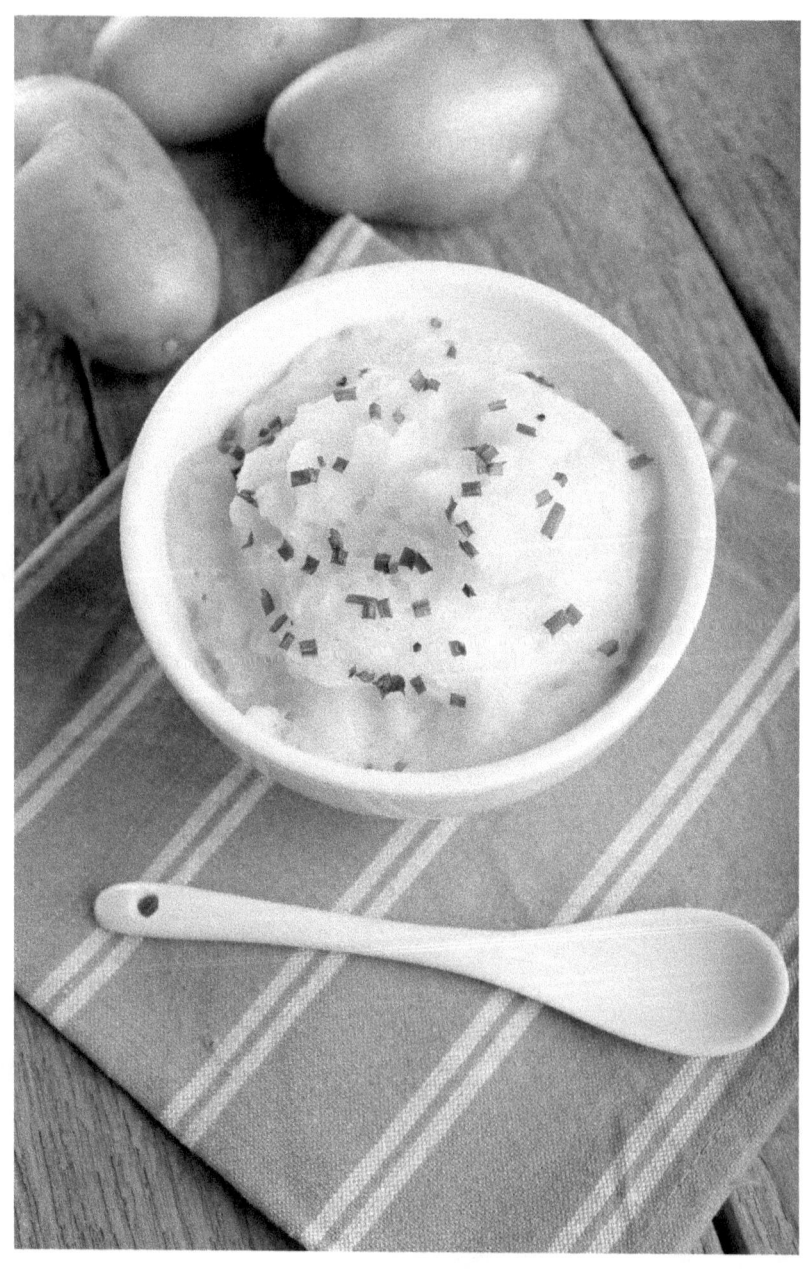

Notes

www.ingramcontent.com/pod-product-compliance
Lightning Source LLC
Chambersburg PA
CBHW070722030426
42336CB00013B/1890